ICD-10

The ICD-10 Classification of Mental and Behavioural Disorders

Diagnostic criteria for research

World Health Organization, Geneva
A.I.T.B.S. Publishers & Distributors (Regd.) Delhi-51

Issued as a publication by the World Health Organization in 2006 under the title The ICD-10 Classification of Mental & Behavioral Disorders, (Clinical Descriptions and Diagnostic Guidelines)

Indian Edition

ISBN 81-7473-237-3 (A.I.T.B.S.)
ISBN 92-4-154455-4 (WHO)

Published by
A.I.T.B.S. Publishers & Distributors (Regd.)
J-5/6, Krishan Nagar, Delhi-110 051 (India)

Printed at Delhi

Contents

Preface	v
Acknowledgements	x
Notes for users	1
ICD-10 Chapter V(F) and associated diagnostic instruments	4
List of categories	5
Diagnostic criteria for research	27
Annex 1. Provisional criteria for selected disorders	173
Annex 2. Culture-specific disorders	176
List of individual experts	189
List of field trial coordinating centres, field trial centres reporting to them, and investigators	191
Index	223

Preface

In the early 1960s, the Mental Health Programme of the World Health Organization (WHO) became actively engaged in a programme aiming to improve the diagnosis and classification of mental disorders. At that time, WHO convened a series of meetings to review knowledge, actively involving representatives of different disciplines, various schools of thought in psychiatry, and all parts of the world in the programme. It stimulated and conducted research on criteria for classification and for reliability of diagnosis, and produced and promulgated procedures for joint rating of videotaped interviews and other useful research methods. Numerous proposals to improve the classification of mental disorders resulted from the extensive consultation process, and these were used in drafting the Eighth Revision of the International Classification of Diseases (ICD-8). A glossary defining each category of mental disorder in ICD-8 was developed. The programme activities also resulted in the establishment of a network of individuals and centres who continued to work on issues related to the improvement of psychiatric classification (*1*, *2*).

The 1970s saw further growth of interest in improving psychiatric classification worldwide. Expansion of international contacts, the undertaking of several international collaborative studies, and the availability of new treatments all contributed to this trend. Several national psychiatric bodies encouraged the development of specific criteria for classification in order to improve diagnostic reliability. In particular, the American Psychiatric Association developed and promulgated its Third Revision of the Diagnostic and Statistical Manual, which incorporated operational criteria into its classification system.

In 1978, WHO entered into a long-term collaborative project with the Alcohol, Drug Abuse, and Mental Health Administration (ADAMHA) in the USA, aiming to facilitate further improvements in the classification and diagnosis of mental disorders, and alcohol- and drug-related problems (*3*). A series of workshops brought together scientists from a number of different psychiatric traditions and cultures, reviewed knowledge in specified areas, and developed recommendations for future research. A major international conference on classification and diagnosis was held in Copenhagen, Denmark, in 1982 to review the recommendations that emerged from these workshops and to outline a research agenda and guidelines for future work (*4*).

Several major research efforts were undertaken to implement the recommendations of the Copenhagen conference. One of them, involving centres in 17 countries, had as its aim the development of the Composite International Diagnostic Interview, an instrument suitable for conducting epidemiological studies of mental disorders in general population groups in different countries (*5, 6*). Another major project focused on developing an assessment instrument suitable for use by clinicians (Schedules for Clinical Assessment in Neuropsychiatry) (*7*). Still another study was initiated to develop an instrument for the assessment of personality disorders in different countries (the International Personality Disorder Examination) (*8*).

In addition, several lexicons have been, or are being, prepared to provide clear definitions of terms (*9*). A mutually beneficial relationship evolved between these projects and the work on definitions of mental and behavioural disorders in the Tenth Revision of the *International Statistical Classification of Diseases and Related Health Problems* (ICD-10) (*10*). Converting diagnostic criteria into diagnostic algorithms incorporated in the assessment instruments was useful in uncovering inconsistencies, ambiguities and overlap and allowing their removal. The work on refining the ICD-10 also helped to shape the assessment instruments. The final result was a clear set of criteria for ICD-10 and assessment instruments which can produce data necessary for the classification of disorders according to the criteria included in Chapter V(F) of ICD-10.

The Copenhagen conference also recommended that the viewpoints of the different psychiatric traditions be presented in publications describing the origins of the classification in the ICD-10. This resulted in several major publications, including a volume that contains a series of presentations highlighting the origins of classification in contemporary psychiatry (*11*).

Clinical descriptions and diagnostic guidelines was the first of a series of publications developed from Chapter V(F) of ICD-10 (*12*). That publication was the culmination of the efforts of numerous people who contributed to it over many years. The work went through several major drafts, each prepared after extensive consultation with panels of experts, national and international psychiatric societies, and individual consultants. The draft in use in 1987 was the basis of field trials conducted in some 40 countries, which constituted the largest ever research effort of its type designed to improve psychiatric diagnosis (*13, 14*). The results of the trials were used in finalizing the clinical guidelines.

The text presented here has also been extensively tested (*15*). A list of the researchers and clinicians involved, in 32 countries, is given at the end of the book, together with a list of people who helped in drafting texts or commented on them. Further texts in the series will include a version for use by general health care workers, a multiaxial presentation of the classification, a series of "fascicles" dealing in more detail with special problems (e.g. the assessment and classification of mental retardation), and "crosswalks" — allowing cross-reference between corresponding terms in ICD-10, ICD-9 and ICD-8 (*15, 16*).

Use of this publication is described in the Notes for Users (page 1). Annex 1 provides suggestions for diagnostic criteria that may be useful in research on several conditions that do not appear as such in the ICD-10 (except as index terms). The Acknowledgements section is of particular significance since it bears witness to the very many individual experts and institutions worldwide who actively participated in the production of the classification of mental and behavioural disorders and the various texts that accompany it. All the major traditions and schools of psychiatry are represented, giving this work a uniquely international character. The classification of mental and behavioural disorders and the guidelines for diagnosis were produced and tested in many languages; the arduous process of ensuring equivalence of translations has resulted in improvements in the clarity, simplicity, and logical structure of the texts in English and in other languages.

The texts based on the ICD-10 classification of mental and behavioural disorders, and the classification itself, are thus a product of collaboration, in the true sense of the word, between many individuals and agencies in numerous countries. They were produced in the hope that they will serve as a strong support to the work of all who are concerned with caring for the mentally ill and their families, worldwide.

Further improvements and simplifications of the classification of mental disorders should become possible as our knowledge increases and experience with the current version accumulates. The task of collecting and digesting comments and results of tests of the classification will remain largely on the shoulders of the centres that collaborated with WHO in the development of the classification. These centres, and their current directors, are listed at the end of the Acknowledgements section: it is hoped that they will continue to be involved in the improvement of the WHO classifications and associated materials in the future and to assist the Organization in this work as generously as they have so far.

Numerous publications have arisen from field trial centres, describing results of their studies in connection with ICD-10. A full list of these publications and reprints of the articles can be obtained on request from Division of Mental Health, World Health Organization, 1211 Geneva 27, Switzerland.

A classification is a way of seeing the world at a point in time. There is no doubt that scientific progress and experience with the use of these research criteria will require their revision and updating. I hope that such revisions will be the product of the same cordial and productive worldwide scientific collaboration as that which has produced the current text.

Norman Sartorius
Director, Division of Mental Health
World Health Organization

References

1. Kramer M et al. The ICD-9 classification of mental disorders: a review of its development and contents. *Acta psychiatrica scandinavica*, 1979, **59**: 241–262.

2. Sartorius N. Classification: an international perspective. *Psychiatric annals*, 1976, **6**: 22–35.

3. Jablensky A et al. Diagnosis and classification of mental disorders and alcohol- and drug-related problems: a research agenda for the 1980s. *Psychological medicine*, 1983, **13**: 907–921.

4. *Mental disorders, alcohol- and drug-related problems: international perspectives on their diagnosis and classification.* Amsterdam, Excerpta Medica, 1985 (International Congress Series, No. 669).

5. Robins L et al. The composite international diagnostic interview. *Archives of general psychiatry*, 1989, **45**: 1069–1077.

6. *Composite International Diagnostic Interview 1.1.* Washington, DC, American Psychiatric Press Inc., 1993.

7. Wing JK et al. SCAN: Schedules for clinical assessment in neuropsychiatry. *Archives of general psychiatry*, 1990, **47**: 589–593.

8. Loranger AW et al. The WHO/ADAMHA International Pilot Study of Personality Disorders: background and purpose. *Journal of personality disorders*, 1991, **5**: 296–306.

9. *Lexicon of psychiatric and mental health terms*, 2nd ed. Geneva, World Health Organization, 1994.

10. *International Statistical Classification of Diseases and Related Health Problems. Tenth Revision*. Geneva, World Health Organization.
Vol. 1: Tabular list, 1992
Vol. 2: Instruction manual, 1993
Vol. 3: Index, 1994

11. Sartorius N et al., eds. *Sources and traditions of classification in psychiatry*. Toronto, Hogrefe and Huber, 1990.

12. *The ICD-10 Classification of Mental and Behavioural Disorders. Clinical descriptions and diagnostic guidelines*. Geneva, World Health Organization, 1992.

13. Sartorius N et al., eds. Psychiatric classification in an international perspective. *British journal of psychiatry*, 1988, **152** (Suppl.).

14. Sartorius N et al. Progress towards achieving a common language in psychiatry: results from the field trials of the clinical guidelines accompanying the WHO Classification of Mental and Behavioural Disorders in ICD-10. *Archives of general psychiatry*, 1993, **50**: 115–124.

15. Sartorius N. The classification of mental disorders in the Tenth Revision of The International Classification of Diseases. *European journal of psychiatry*, 1991, **6**: 315–322.

16. *The ICD-10 Classification of Mental and Behavioural Disorders: Conversion tables between ICD-8, ICD-9 and ICD-10*. Geneva, World Health Organization, 1992 (unpublished WHO document WHO/MNH/92.16, available on request from Division of Mental Health, World Health Organization, 1211 Geneva 27, Switzerland).

Acknowledgements

Many individuals and organizations have contributed to the production of the classification of mental and behavioural disorders in ICD-10 and to the development of the texts that accompany it. The Acknowledgements section of *Clinical descriptions and diagnostic guidelines*[1] contains a list of researchers and clinicians in some 40 countries who participated in the trials of that document. A similar list is provided on pages 192–222 of this work. Although it is clearly impossible to list all those who have helped in the production of the texts and in their testing, every effort has been made to include at least all those whose contributions were central to the creation of the documents that make up the ICD-10 "family" of classifications and guidelines (see pages 189–190).

Dr A. Jablensky, then Senior Medical Officer in the Division of Mental Health of WHO in Geneva, coordinated the first part of the programme, and thus made a major contribution to the development of the proposals for the text of the criteria. After the proposals for the classification had been assembled and circulated for comment to WHO expert panels and many other individuals, an amended version of the classification was produced for field tests. Tests were conducted according to a protocol produced by WHO staff with the help of Dr J.E. Cooper and other consultants mentioned below, and involved a large number of centres whose work was coordinated by field trial coordinating centres. The coordinating centres, listed below and on pages 192–222, also undertook the task of producing equivalent versions of *Diagnostic criteria for research* in the languages used in their countries.

Dr N. Sartorius had overall responsiblity for the work on the classification of mental and behavioural disorders in ICD-10 and for the production of accompanying documents.

Throughout the work on the ICD-10 documents, Dr J.E. Cooper acted as chief consultant to the project and provided invaluable guidance and help to the WHO coordinating team. Among the team members were Dr J. van Drimmelen, who has

[1] *The ICD-10 Classification of Mental and Behavioural Disorders. Clinical descriptions and diagnostic guidelines*. Geneva, World Health Organization, 1992.

worked with WHO from the beginning of the process of developing ICD-10 proposals; Dr B. Üstün, who has made particularly valuable contributions during the field trials of the criteria and the analysis of the data they produced; Mr A. L'Hours, Technical Officer, Strengthening of Epidemiological and Statistical Services, who provided generous support, ensuring compliance between the ICD-10 development in general and the production of this classification; Mrs J. Wilson, who conscientiously and efficiently handled the innumerable administrative tasks linked to the field tests and other activities related to the project; and Mrs Ruthbeth Finerman, Associate Professor in anthropology, who provided the information upon which Annex 2, Culture-specific disorders, is based.

A number of other consultants, including in particular Dr A. Bertelsen, Dr H. Dilling, Dr J. López-Ibor, Dr C. Pull, Dr D. Regier, Dr M. Rutter and Dr N. Wig, were also closely involved in this work, functioning not only as heads of field trial coordinating centres but also providing advice and guidance about issues in their areas of expertise and relevant to the psychiatric traditions of the groups of countries about which they are particularly knowledgeable.

Among the agencies whose help was of vital importance was the Alcohol, Drug Abuse, and Mental Health Administration (now National Institutes of Health) in the USA, which provided generous support to the activities preparatory to the drafting of ICD-10, and which ensured effective and productive consultation between groups working on ICD-10 and those working on the fourth revision of the Diagnostic and Statistical Manual (DSM-IV) classification of the American Psychiatric Association (APA). Close direct collaboration with the chairmen and the working groups of the APA Task Force on DSM-IV chaired by Dr A. Frances allowed an extensive exchange of views and helped in ensuring compatibility between the texts. Invaluable help was also provided by the WHO Advisory Committee on ICD-10, chaired by the late Dr E. Strömgren; the World Psychiatric Association and its special committee on classification, the World Federation for Mental Health, the World Association for Psychosocial Rehabilitation, the World Association of Social Psychiatry, the World Federation of Neurology, the International Union of Psychological Societies, and the WHO Collaborating Centres for Research and Training in Mental Health, located in some 40 countries, were particularly useful in the collection of commments and suggestions from their parts of the world.

Governments of WHO Member States, including in particular Belgium, Germany, the Netherlands, Spain, and the USA, also provided direct support to the process of developing the classification of mental and behavioural disorders, both through their designated contributions to WHO and through contributions and financial support to the centres that participated in this work.

Field trial coordinating centres and directors

Dr A. Bertelsen, Institute of Psychiatric Demography, Psychiatric Hospital, University of Aarhus, Risskov, Denmark

Dr D. Caetano, Department of Psychiatry, State University of Campinas, Campinas, Brazil

Dr S. Channabasavanna, National Institute of Mental Health and Neurosciences, Bangalore, India

Dr H. Dilling, Psychiatric Clinic of the Medical School, Lübeck, Germany

Dr M. Gelder, Department of Psychiatry, Oxford University Hospital, Warneford Hospital, Headington, England

Dr D. Kemali, Institute of Psychiatry, First Faculty of Medicine, University of Naples, Naples, Italy

Dr J.J. López-Ibor Jr, López-Ibor Clinic, Puerto de Hierro, Madrid, Spain

Dr G. Mellsop, The Wellington Clinical School, Wellington Hospital, Wellington, New Zealand

Dr Y. Nakane, Department of Neuropsychiatry, Nagasaki University, School of Medicine, Nagasaki, Japan

Dr A. Okasha, Department of Psychiatry, Ain-Shams University, Cairo, Egypt

Dr C. Pull, Department of Neuropsychiatry, Centre Hospitalier de Luxembourg, Luxembourg, Luxembourg

Dr D. Regier, Division of Clinical Research, National Institute of Mental Health, Rockville, MD, USA

Dr S. Tzirkin, All Union Research Centre of Mental Health, Institute of Psychiatry, Academy of Medical Sciences, Moscow, Russian Federation

Dr Xu Tao-Yuan, Department of Psychiatry, Shanghai Psychiatric Hospital, Shanghai, China

Former directors of field trial coordinating centres

Dr J.E. Cooper, Department of Psychiatry, Queen's Medical Centre, Nottingham, England

Dr R. Takahashi, Department of Psychiatry, Tokyo Medical and Dental University, Tokyo, Japan

Dr N. Wig, Regional Adviser for Mental Health, World Health Organization, Regional Office for the Eastern Mediterranean, Alexandria, Egypt

Dr Yang De-Sen, Hunan Medical College, Changsha, Hunan, China

Notes for users

1. The content of *Diagnostic criteria for research* (DCR-10) is derived from Chapter V(F), Mental and behavioural disorders, of ICD-10. It provides specific criteria for the diagnoses contained in *Clinical descriptions and diagnostic guidelines* (CDDG), which was produced for general clinical and educational use by psychiatrists and other mental health professionals.[1]

2. Although completely compatible with both CDDG and Chapter V(F) of ICD-10, DCR-10 has a somewhat different style and layout. It is not designed to be used alone, and researchers should therefore make themselves familiar with CDDG. DCR-10 does not contain the descriptions of the clinical concepts upon which the research criteria are based, or any comments on commonly associated features which, although not essential for diagnosis, may well be relevant for both clinicians and researchers. These features are to be found in CDDG, the introductory chapters of which also contain information and comments that are relevant for both clinical and research uses of ICD-10. It is presumed that anyone using DCR-10 will have a copy of CDDG.

3. Certain other differences between DCR-10 and CDDG should be appreciated before DCR-10 can be used satisfactorily.

   (a) Like other published diagnostic criteria for research, the criteria of DCR-10 are deliberately restrictive: their use allows the selection of groups of individuals whose symptoms and other characteristics resemble each other in clearly stated ways. This tends to maximize the homogeneity of groups of patients but limits the generalizations that can be made. Researchers wishing to study the overlap of disorders or the best way to define boundaries between them may therefore need to supplement the criteria so as to allow the inclusion of atypical cases.

   (b) It is never appropriate to provide detailed criteria for the "unspecified" (.9) categories of the overall ICD-10 (Chapter V(F)) classification, and rarely appropriate for the "other" (.8) categories. Annex 1 (page 173) provides suggestions for criteria for some of the few exceptions; place-

[1] *The ICD-10 Classification of Mental and Behavioural Disorders. Clinical descriptions and diagnostic guidelines*. Geneva, World Health Organization, 1992.

ment of these criteria in an annex implies that their present status is somewhat controversial or tentative and that further research is to be encouraged.

(c) Similarly, there is no requirement for extensive rules on mutual exclusions and co-morbidity in a set of diagnostic criteria for research, since different research projects have varied requirements for these, depending upon their objectives. Some of the more obvious and frequently used exclusion clauses have been included in DCR-10 as a reminder and for the convenience of users; more can be found in CDDG if required.

4. As a general rule, interference with the performance of social roles has not been used as a diagnostic criterion in ICD-10. This rule has been followed in DCR-10 as far as possible, but there are a few unavoidable exceptions, the most obvious being simple schizophrenia and dissocial personality disorder. Once the decision had been made to include these disorders in the classification, it was considered best to do so without modifying the concepts; as a consequence it became necessary to include interference with social role in the diagnostic criteria for these disorders. Experience and further research should show whether these decisions were justified.

   For many of the disorders of childhood and adolescence, some form of interference with social behaviour and relationships is included among the diagnostic criteria. Initially, this appears to contravene the general ICD rule mentioned above. However, close examination of the disturbances classified in F80–F89 and F90–F98 shows that the need for social criteria is occasioned by the more complicated and interactive nature of the subject matter. Children often show general misery and frustration, but rarely produce specific complaints and symptoms equivalent to those that characterize the disorders of adults. Many of the disorders in F80–F89 and F90–F98 are joint disturbances that can be described only by indicating how roles within the family, school, or peer group are affected.

5. For the same reasons given in 3(c) above, definitions of remission, relapse, and duration of episodes have been provided in DCR-10 in only a limited number of instances. Further suggestions will be found in the lexicon of terms to Chapter V(F) of ICD-10.[1]

[1] *Lexicon of psychiatric and mental health terms*, 2nd ed. Geneva, World Health Organization, 1994.

6. The criteria are labelled with letters and/or numbers to indicate their place in a hierarchy of generality and importance. General criteria, which *must* be fulfilled by all members of a group of disorders (such as the general criteria for all varieties of dementia, or for the main types of schizophrenia) are labelled with a capital G, plus a number. Obligatory criteria for individual disorders are distinguished by capital letters alone (A, B, C, etc.). Numbers (1, 2, 3, etc.) and lower case letters (a, b, etc.) are used to identify further groups and sub-groups of characteristics, of which only some are required for the diagnosis. To avoid the use of "and/or", when it is specified that *either* of two criteria is required, it is always assumed that the presence of *both* criteria also satisfies the requirement.

7. When DCR-10 is used in research on patients who also suffer from neurological disorders, researchers may also wish to use the neurological application of ICD-10 (ICD-10NA)[1] and the accompanying glossary (in preparation).

8. The two annexes to DCR-10 are concerned with disorders of uncertain or provisional status. Annex 1 deals with some affective disorders that have been the subject of recent research, and certain personality disorders. Although the concepts are regarded as clinically useful in some countries, the disorders themselves are of uncertain status from an international viewpoint; it is hoped that their inclusion here will encourage research concerning their usefulness.

   Annex 2 provides provisional descriptions of a number of disorders that are often referred to as "culture-specific". There are grounds for supposing that they might be better regarded as cultural variants of disorders already present in ICD-10 Chapter V(F), but reliable and detailed clinical information is still too scanty to allow definite conclusions to be drawn about them. The considerable practical difficulties involved in field studies of individuals with these disorders are recognized, but inclusion of the descriptions in DCR-10 may stimulate research by workers who are familiar with the languages and cultures of those affected. Information in Annex 2 will be supplemented by that in a lexicon of terms used in cross-cultural psychiatry that is expected to become available in 1994.

9. Note that "and" in category titles stands for "and/or".

[1] *Application of the International Classification of Diseases to Neurology.* Geneva, World Health Organization (in preparation).

ICD-10 Chapter V(F) and associated diagnostic instruments

The Schedule for Clinical Assessment in Neuropsychiatry (SCAN), the Composite International Diagnostic Interview (CIDI), and the International Personality Disorder Examination (IPDE) have been developed within the framework of the WHO/ADAMHA Joint Project on Diagnosis and Classification of Mental Disorders, Alcohol- and Drug-related Problems. More information about these instruments can be obtained from the Division of Mental Health, World Health Organization, 1211 Geneva 27, Switzerland.

Training in the use of these instruments can at present be obtained in the following languages: Chinese, Danish, Dutch, English, French, German, Greek, Hindi, Kannada, Portuguese, Spanish, Tamil, and Turkish.

List of categories

F00 – F09
Organic, including symptomatic, mental disorders

F00 Dementia in Alzheimer's disease

F00.0 Dementia in Alzheimer's disease with early onset
F00.1 Dementia in Alzheimer's disease with late onset
F00.2 Dementia in Alzheimer's disease, atypical or mixed type
F00.9 Dementia in Alzheimer's disease, unspecified

F01 Vascular dementia

F01.0 Vascular dementia of acute onset
F01.1 Multi-infarct dementia
F01.2 Subcortical vascular dementia
F01.3 Mixed cortical and subcortical vascular dementia
F01.8 Other vascular dementia
F01.9 Vascular dementia, unspecified

F02 Dementia in other diseases classified elsewhere

F02.0 Dementia in Pick's disease
F02.1 Dementia in Creutzfeldt–Jakob disease
F02.2 Dementia in Huntington's disease
F02.3 Dementia in Parkinson's disease
F02.4 Dementia in human immunodeficiency virus [HIV] disease
F02.8 Dementia in other specified diseases classified elsewhere

F03 Unspecified dementia

A fifth character may be used to specify dementia in F00–F03, as follows:

*.x*0 Without additional symptoms
*.x*1 With other symptoms, predominantly delusional
*.x*2 With other symptoms, predominantly hallucinatory
*.x*3 With other symptoms, predominantly depressive
*.x*4 With other mixed symptoms

A sixth character may be used to indicate the severity of the dementia:

.*xx*0 Mild
.*xx*1 Moderate
.*xx*2 Severe

F04 Organic amnesic syndrome, not induced by alcohol and other psychoactive substances

F05 Delirium, not induced by alcohol and other psychoactive substances

F05.0 Delirium, not superimposed on dementia, so described
F05.1 Delirium, superimposed on dementia
F05.8 Other delirium
F05.9 Delirium, unspecified

F06 Other mental disorders due to brain damage and dysfunction and to physical disease

F06.0 Organic hallucinosis
F06.1 Organic catatonic disorder
F06.2 Organic delusional [schizophrenia-like] disorder
F06.3 Organic mood [affective] disorder
.30 Organic manic disorder
.31 Organic bipolar disorder
.32 Organic depressive disorder
.33 Organic mixed affective disorder
F06.4 Organic anxiety disorder
F06.5 Organic dissociative disorder
F06.6 Organic emotionally labile [asthenic] disorder
F06.7 Mild cognitive disorder
.70 Not associated with a physical disorder
.71 Associated with a physical disorder
F06.8 Other specified mental disorders due to brain damage and dysfunction and to physical disease
F06.9 Unspecified mental disorder due to brain damage and dysfunction and to physical disease

F07 Personality and behavioural disorders due to brain disease, damage and dysfunction

F07.0 Organic personality disorder
F07.1 Postencephalitic syndrome
F07.2 Postconcussional syndrome

F07.8 Other organic personality and behavioural disorders due to brain disease, damage and dysfunction

F07.9 Unspecified mental disorder due to brain disease, damage and dysfunction

F09 Unspecified organic or symptomatic mental disorder

F10 – F19
Mental and behavioural disorders due to psychoactive substance use

F10.– Mental and behavioural disorders due to use of alcohol

F11.– Mental and behavioural disorders due to use of opioids

F12.– Mental and behavioural disorders due to use of cannabinoids

F13.– Mental and behavioural disorders due to use of sedatives or hypnotics

F14.– Mental and behavioural disorders due to use of cocaine

F15.– Mental and behavioural disorders due to use of other stimulants, including caffeine

F16.– Mental and behavioural disorders due to use of hallucinogens

F17.– Mental and behavioural disorders due to use of tobacco

F18.– Mental and behavioural disorders due to use of volatile solvents

F19.– Mental and behavioural disorders due to multiple drug use and use of other psychoactive substances

Four-, five- and six-character categories are used to specify the clinical conditions as follows, and diagnostic criteria particular to each psychoactive substance are provided where appropriate for acute intoxication and withdrawal state:

F1*x*.0 Acute intoxication
- .00 Uncomplicated
- .01 With trauma or other bodily injury
- .02 With other medical complications
- .03 With delirium
- .04 With perceptual distortions
- .05 With coma
- .06 With convulsions
- .07 Pathological intoxication

F1*x*.1 Harmful use

F1*x*.2 Dependence syndrome
- .20 Currently abstinent
  - .200 Early remission
  - .201 Partial remission
  - .202 Full remission
- .21 Currently abstinent, but in a protected environment
- .22 Currently on a clinically supervised maintenance or replacement regime [controlled dependence]
- .23 Currently abstinent, but receiving treatment with aversive or blocking drugs
- .24 Currently using the substance [active dependence]
  - .240 Without physical features
  - .241 With physical features
- .25 Continuous use
- .26 Episodic use [dipsomania]

F1*x*.3 Withdrawal state
- .30 Uncomplicated
- .31 With convulsions

F1*x*.4 Withdrawal state with delirium
- .40 Without convulsions
- .41 With convulsions

F1*x*.5 Psychotic disorder
- .50 Schizophrenia-like
- .51 Predominantly delusional
- .52 Predominantly hallucinatory
- .53 Predominantly polymorphic
- .54 Predominantly depressive psychotic symptoms
- .55 Predominantly manic psychotic symptoms
- .56 Mixed

F1*x*.6 Amnesic syndrome

F1*x*.7 Residual and late-onset psychotic disorder
- .70 Flashbacks
- .71 Personality or behaviour disorder
- .72 Residual affective disorder
- .73 Dementia

.74 Other persisting cognitive disorder
.75 Late-onset psychotic disorder

F1*x*.8 Other mental and behavioural disorders

F1*x*.9 Unspecified mental and behavioural disorder

F20 – F29
Schizophrenia, schizotypal and delusional disorders

F20 Schizophrenia

F20.0 Paranoid schizophrenia
F20.1 Hebephrenic schizophrenia
F20.2 Catatonic schizophrenia
F20.3 Undifferentiated schizophrenia
F20.4 Post-schizophrenic depression
F20.5 Residual schizophrenia
F20.6 Simple schizophrenia
F20.8 Other schizophrenia
F20.9 Schizophrenia, unspecified

A fifth character may be used to classify course:

.*x*0 Continuous
.*x*1 Episodic with progressive deficit
.*x*2 Episodic with stable deficit
.*x*3 Episodic remittent
.*x*4 Incomplete remission
.*x*5 Complete remission
.*x*8 Other
.*x*9 Course uncertain, period of observation too short

F21 Schizotypal disorder

F22 Persistent delusional disorders

F22.0 Delusional disorder
F22.8 Other persistent delusional disorders
F22.9 Persistent delusional disorder, unspecified

F23 Acute and transient psychotic disorders

F23.0 Acute polymorphic psychotic disorder without symptoms of schizophrenia
F23.1 Acute polymorphic psychotic disorder with symptoms of schizophrenia
F23.2 Acute schizophrenia-like psychotic disorder
F23.3 Other acute predominantly delusional psychotic disorder
F23.8 Other acute and transient psychotic disorders
F23.9 Acute and transient psychotic disorder, unspecified

A fifth character may be used to identify the presence or absence of associated acute stress:

.x0 Without associated acute stress
.x1 With associated acute stress

F24 Induced delusional disorder

F25 Schizoaffective disorders

F25.0 Schizoaffective disorder, manic type
F25.1 Schizoaffective disorder, depressive type
F25.2 Schizoaffective disorder, mixed type
F25.8 Other schizoaffective disorders
F25.9 Schizoaffective disorder, unspecified

A fifth character may be used to classify the following subtypes:

.x0 Concurrent affective and schizophrenic symptoms only
.x1 Concurrent affective and schizophrenic symptoms, plus persistence of the schizophrenic symptoms beyond the duration of the affective symptoms

F28 Other nonorganic psychotic disorders

F29 Unspecified nonorganic psychosis

F30 – F39
Mood [affective] disorders

F30 Manic episode

F30.0 Hypomania
F30.1 Mania without psychotic symptoms
F30.2 Mania with psychotic symptoms
.20 With mood-congruent psychotic symptoms
.21 With mood-incongruent psychotic symptoms
F30.8 Other manic episodes
F30.9 Manic episode, unspecified

F31 Bipolar affective disorder

F31.0 Bipolar affective disorder, current episode hypomanic
F31.1 Bipolar affective disorder, current episode manic without psychotic symptoms
F31.2 Bipolar affective disorder, current episode manic with psychotic symptoms
.20 With mood-congruent psychotic symptoms
.21 With mood-incongruent psychotic symptoms
F31.3 Bipolar affective disorder, current episode mild or moderate depression
.30 Without somatic syndrome
.31 With somatic syndrome
F31.4 Bipolar affective disorder, current episode severe depression without psychotic symptoms
F31.5 Bipolar affective disorder, current episode severe depression with psychotic symptoms
.50 With mood-congruent psychotic symptoms
.51 With mood-incongruent psychotic symptoms
F31.6 Bipolar affective disorder, current episode mixed
F31.7 Bipolar affective disorder, currently in remission
F31.8 Other bipolar affective disorders
F31.9 Bipolar affective disorder, unspecified

F32 Depressive episode

F32.0 Mild depressive episode
.00 Without somatic syndrome
.01 With somatic syndrome
F32.1 Moderate depressive episode
.10 Without somatic syndrome
.11 With somatic syndrome

F32.2 Severe depressive episode without psychotic symptoms
F32.3 Severe depressive episode with psychotic symptoms
.30 With mood-congruent psychotic symptoms
.31 With mood-incongruent psychotic symptoms
F32.8 Other depressive episodes
F32.9 Depressive episode, unspecified

F33 Recurrent depressive disorder
F33.0 Recurrent depressive disorder, current episode mild
.00 Without somatic syndrome
.01 With somatic syndrome
F33.1 Recurrent depressive disorder, current episode moderate
.10 Without somatic syndrome
.11 With somatic syndrome
F33.2 Recurrent depressive disorder, current episode severe without psychotic symptoms
F33.3 Recurrent depressive disorder, current episode severe with psychotic symptoms
.30 With mood-congruent psychotic symptoms
.31 With mood-incongruent psychotic symptoms
F33.4 Recurrent depressive disorder, currently in remission
F33.8 Other recurrent depressive disorders
F33.9 Recurrent depressive disorder, unspecified

F34 Persistent mood [affective] disorders
F34.0 Cyclothymia
F34.1 Dysthymia
F34.8 Other persistent mood [affective] disorders
F34.9 Persistent mood [affective] disorder, unspecified

F38 Other mood [affective] disorders
F38.0 Other single mood [affective] disorders
.00 Mixed affective episode
F38.1 Other recurrent mood [affective] disorders
.10 Recurrent brief depressive disorder
F38.8 Other specified mood [affective] disorders

F39 Unspecified mood [affective] disorder

F40 – F48
Neurotic, stress-related and somatoform disorders

F40 Phobic anxiety disorders

F40.0 Agoraphobia
.00 Without panic disorder
.01 With panic disorder
F40.1 Social phobias
F40.2 Specific (isolated) phobias
F40.8 Other phobic anxiety disorders
F40.9 Phobic anxiety disorder, unspecified

F41 Other anxiety disorders

F41.0 Panic disorder [episodic paroxysmal anxiety]
.00 Moderate
.01 Severe
F41.1 Generalized anxiety disorder
F41.2 Mixed anxiety and depressive disorder
F41.3 Other mixed anxiety disorders
F41.8 Other specified anxiety disorders
F41.9 Anxiety disorder, unspecified

F42 Obsessive–compulsive disorder

F42.0 Predominantly obsessional thoughts or ruminations
F42.1 Predominantly compulsive acts [obsessional rituals]
F42.2 Mixed obsessional thoughts and acts
F42.8 Other obsessive–compulsive disorders
F42.9 Obsessive–compulsive disorder, unspecified

F43 Reaction to severe stress, and adjustment disorders

F43.0 Acute stress reaction
.00 Mild
.01 Moderate
.02 Severe
F43.1 Post-traumatic stress disorder
F43.2 Adjustment disorders
.20 Brief depressive reaction
.21 Prolonged depressive reaction
.22 Mixed anxiety and depressive reaction
.23 With predominant disturbance of other emotions
.24 With predominant disturbance of conduct

.25 With mixed disturbance of emotions and conduct
.28 With other specified predominant symptoms
F43.8 Other reactions to severe stress
F43.9 Reaction to severe stress, unspecified

F44 Dissociative [conversion] disorders
F44.0 Dissociative amnesia
F44.1 Dissociative fugue
F44.2 Dissociative stupor
F44.3 Trance and possession disorders
F44.4 Dissociative motor disorders
F44.5 Dissociative convulsions
F44.6 Dissociative anaesthesia and sensory loss
F44.7 Mixed dissociative [conversion] disorders
F44.8 Other dissociative [conversion] disorders
.80 Ganser's syndrome
.81 Multiple personality disorder
.82 Transient dissociative [conversion] disorders occurring in childhood and adolescence
.88 Other specified dissociative [conversion] disorders
F44.9 Dissociative [conversion] disorder, unspecified

F45 Somatoform disorders
F45.0 Somatization disorder
F45.1 Undifferentiated somatoform disorder
F45.2 Hypochondriacal disorders
F45.3 Somatoform autonomic dysfunction
.30 Heart and cardiovascular system
.31 Upper gastrointestinal tract
.32 Lower gastrointestinal tract
.33 Respiratory system
.34 Genitourinary system
.38 Other organ or system
F45.4 Persistent somatoform pain disorder
F45.8 Other somatoform disorders
F45.9 Somatoform disorder, unspecified

F48 Other neurotic disorders
F48.0 Neurasthenia
F48.1 Depersonalization–derealization syndrome
F48.8 Other specified neurotic disorders
F48.9 Neurotic disorder, unspecified

F50 – F59
Behavioural syndromes associated with physiological disturbances and physical factors

F50 Eating disorders

F50.0 Anorexia nervosa
F50.1 Atypical anorexia nervosa
F50.2 Bulimia nervosa
F50.3 Atypical bulimia nervosa
F50.4 Overeating associated with other psychological disturbances
F50.5 Vomiting associated with other psychological disturbances
F50.8 Other eating disorders
F50.9 Eating disorder, unspecified

F51 Nonorganic sleep disorders

F51.0 Nonorganic insomnia
F51.1 Nonorganic hypersomnia
F51.2 Nonorganic disorder of the sleep–wake schedule
F51.3 Sleepwalking [somnambulism]
F51.4 Sleep terrors [night terrors]
F51.5 Nightmares
F51.8 Other nonorganic sleep disorders
F51.9 Nonorganic sleep disorder, unspecified

F52 Sexual dysfunction, not caused by organic disorder or disease

F52.0 Lack or loss of sexual desire
F52.1 Sexual aversion and lack of sexual enjoyment
.10 Sexual aversion
.11 Lack of sexual enjoyment
F52.2 Failure of genital response
F52.3 Orgasmic dysfunction
F52.4 Premature ejaculation
F52.5 Nonorganic vaginismus
F52.6 Nonorganic dyspareunia
F52.7 Excessive sexual drive
F52.8 Other sexual dysfunction, not caused by organic disorder or disease
F52.9 Unspecified sexual dysfunction, not caused by organic disorder or disease

F53 Mental and behavioural disorders associated with the puerperium, not elsewhere classified

F53.0 Mild mental and behavioural disorders associated with the puerperium, not elsewhere classified

F53.1 Severe mental and behavioural disorders associated with the puerperium, not elsewhere classified

F53.8 Other mental and behavioural disorders associated with the puerperium, not elsewhere classified

F53.9 Puerperal mental disorder, unspecified

F54 Psychological and behavioural factors associated with disorders or diseases classified elsewhere

F55 Abuse of non-dependence-producing substances

F55.0 Antidepressants
F55.1 Laxatives
F55.2 Analgesics
F55.3 Antacids
F55.4 Vitamins
F55.5 Steroids or hormones
F55.6 Specific herbal or folk remedies
F55.8 Other substances that do not produce dependence
F55.9 Unspecified

F59 Unspecified behavioural syndromes associated with physiological disturbances and physical factors

F60 – F69
Disorders of adult personality and behaviour

F60 Specific personality disorders

F60.0 Paranoid personality disorder
F60.1 Schizoid personality disorder
F60.2 Dissocial personality disorder
F60.3 Emotionally unstable personality disorder
.30 Impulsive type
.31 Borderline type
F60.4 Histrionic personality disorder
F60.5 Anankastic personality disorder
F60.6 Anxious [avoidant] personality disorder
F60.7 Dependent personality disorder
F60.8 Other specific personality disorders
F60.9 Personality disorder, unspecified

F61 Mixed and other personality disorders

F61.0 Mixed personality disorder
F61.1 Troublesome personality changes

F62 Enduring personality changes, not attributable to brain damage and disease

F62.0 Enduring personality change after catastrophic experience
F62.1 Enduring personality change after psychiatric illness
F62.8 Other enduring personality changes
F62.9 Enduring personality change, unspecified

F63 Habit and impulse disorders

F63.0 Pathological gambling
F63.1 Pathological fire-setting [pyromania]
F63.2 Pathological stealing [kleptomania]
F63.3 Trichotillomania
F63.8 Other habit and impulse disorders
F63.9 Habit and impulse disorder, unspecified

F64 Gender identity disorders

F64.0 Transsexualism
F64.1 Dual-role transvestism
F64.2 Gender identity disorder of childhood
F64.8 Other gender identity disorders
F64.9 Gender identity disorder, unspecified

F65 Disorders of sexual preference

F65.0 Fetishism
F65.1 Fetishistic transvestism
F65.2 Exhibitionism
F65.3 Voyeurism
F65.4 Paedophilia
F65.5 Sadomasochism
F65.6 Multiple disorders of sexual preference
F65.8 Other disorders of sexual preference
F65.9 Disorder of sexual preference, unspecified

F66 Psychological and behavioural disorders associated with sexual development and orientation

F66.0 Sexual maturation disorder
F66.1 Egodystonic sexual orientation
F66.2 Sexual relationship disorder
F66.8 Other psychosexual development disorders
F66.9 Psychosexual development disorder, unspecified

F68 Other disorders of adult personality and behaviour

F68.0 Elaboration of physical symptoms for psychological reasons
F68.1 Intentional production or feigning of symptoms or disabilities, either physical or psychological [factitious disorder]
F68.8 Other specified disorders of adult personality and behaviour

F69 Unspecified disorder of adult personality and behaviour

F70 – F79
Mental retardation

F70 Mild mental retardation

F71 Moderate mental retardation

F72 Severe mental retardation

F73 Profound mental retardation

F78 Other mental retardation

F79 Unspecified mental retardation

A fourth character may be used to specify the extent of associated impairment of behaviour:

F7*x*.0 No, or minimal, impairment of behaviour
F7*x*.1 Significant impairment of behaviour requiring attention or treatment
F7*x*.2 Other impairments of behaviour
F7*x*.3 Without mention of impairment of behaviour

F80 – F89
Disorders of psychological development

F80 Specific developmental disorders of speech and language

F80.0 Specific speech articulation disorder
F80.1 Expressive language disorder
F80.2 Receptive language disorder
F80.3 Acquired aphasia with epilepsy [Landau–Kleffner syndrome]
F80.8 Other developmental disorders of speech and language
F80.9 Developmental disorder of speech and language, unspecified

F81 Specific developmental disorders of scholastic skills

F81.0 Specific reading disorder
F81.1 Specific spelling disorder
F81.2 Specific disorder of arithmetical skills
F81.3 Mixed disorder of scholastic skills
F81.8 Other developmental disorders of scholastic skills
F81.9 Developmental disorder of scholastic skills, unspecified

F82 Specific developmental disorder of motor function

F83 Mixed specific developmental disorder

F84 Pervasive developmental disorders

F84.0 Childhood autism
F84.1 Atypical autism
.10 Atypicality in age of onset
.11 Atypicality in symptomatology
.12 Atypicality in both age of onset and symptomatology
F84.2 Rett's syndrome
F84.3 Other childhood disintegrative disorder
F84.4 Overactive disorder associated with mental retardation and stereotyped movements
F84.5 Asperger's syndrome
F84.8 Other pervasive developmental disorders
F84.9 Pervasive developmental disorder, unspecified

F88 Other disorders of psychological development

F89 Unspecified disorder of psychological development

F90 – F98
Behavioural and emotional disorders with onset usually occurring in childhood and adolescence

F90 Hyperkinetic disorder
- F90.0 Disturbance of activity and attention
- F90.1 Hyperkinetic conduct disorder
- F90.8 Other hyperkinetic disorders
- F90.9 Hyperkinetic disorder, unspecified

F91 Conduct disorders
- F91.0 Conduct disorder confined to the family context
- F91.1 Unsocialized conduct disorder
- F91.2 Socialized conduct disorder
- F91.3 Oppositional defiant disorder
- F91.8 Other conduct disorders
- F91.9 Conduct disorder, unspecified

F92 Mixed disorders of conduct and emotions
- F92.0 Depressive conduct disorder
- F92.8 Other mixed disorders of conduct and emotions
- F92.9 Mixed disorder of conduct and emotions, unspecified

F93 Emotional disorders with onset specific to childhood
- F93.0 Separation anxiety disorder of childhood
- F93.1 Phobic anxiety disorder of childhood
- F93.2 Social anxiety disorder of childhood
- F93.3 Sibling rivalry disorder
- F93.8 Other childhood emotional disorders
  - .80 Generalized anxiety disorder of childhood
- F93.9 Childhood emotional disorder, unspecified

F94 Disorders of social functioning with onset specific to childhood and adolescence
- F94.0 Elective mutism
- F94.1 Reactive attachment disorder of childhood
- F94.2 Disinhibited attachment disorder of childhood
- F94.8 Other childhood disorders of social functioning
- F94.9 Childhood disorder of social functioning, unspecified

F95 Tic disorders

F95.0 Transient tic disorders
F95.1 Chronic motor or vocal tic disorder
F95.2 Combined vocal and multiple motor tic disorder [de la Tourette's syndrome]
F95.8 Other tic disorders
F95.9 Tic disorder, unspecified

F98 Other behavioural and emotional disorders with onset usually occurring in childhood and adolescence

F98.0 Nonorganic enuresis
- .00 Nocturnal enuresis only
- .01 Diurnal enuresis only
- .02 Nocturnal and diurnal enureses

F98.1 Nonorganic encopresis
- .10 Failure to acquire physiological bowel control
- .11 Adequate bowel control with normal faeces deposited in inappropriate places
- .12 Soiling that is associated with excessively fluid faeces such as with retention with overflow

F98.2 Feeding disorder of infancy and childhood
F98.3 Pica of infancy and childhood
F98.4 Stereotyped movement disorders
- .40 Non-self-injurious
- .41 Self-injurious
- .42 Mixed

F98.5 Stuttering [stammering]
F98.6 Cluttering
F98.8 Other specified behavioural and emotional disorders with onset usually occurring in childhood and adolescence
F98.9 Unspecified behavioural and emotional disorders with onset usually occurring in childhood and adolescence

F99
Unspecified mental disorder

F99 Mental disorder, not otherwise specified

Diagnostic criteria for research

Diagnostic criteria for research

F00 – F09
Organic, including symptomatic, mental disorders

Dementia

G1. There is evidence of each of the following:

(1) A decline in memory, which is most evident in the learning of new information although, in more severe cases, the recall of previously learned information may also be affected. The impairment applies to both verbal and non-verbal material. The decline should be objectively verified by obtaining a reliable history from an informant, supplemented, if possible, by neuropsychological tests or quantified cognitive assessments. The severity of the decline, with mild impairment as the threshold for diagnosis, should be assessed as follows:

Mild. The degree of memory loss is sufficient to interfere with everyday activities, though not so severe as to be incompatible with independent living. The main function affected is the learning of new material. For example, the individual has difficulty in registering, storing, and recalling elements involved in daily living, such as where belongings have been put, social arrangements, or information recently imparted by family members.

Moderate. The degree of memory loss represents a serious handicap to independent living. Only highly learned or very familiar material is retained. New information is retained only occasionally and very briefly. Individuals are unable to recall basic information about their own local geography, what they have recently been doing, or the names of familiar people.

Severe. The degree of memory loss is characterized by the complete inability to retain new information. Only fragments of previously learned information remain. The individual fails to recognize even close relatives.

(2) A decline in other cognitive abilities characterized by deterioration in judgement and thinking, such as planning and organizing, and in the general processing of information. Evidence for this should ideally be obtained from an informant and supplemented, if possible, by neuropsychological tests or quantified objective assessments. Deterioration from a previously higher level of performance should be established.

The severity of the decline, with mild impairment as the threshold for diagnosis, should be assessed as follows:

Mild. The decline in cognitive abilities causes impaired performance in daily living, but not to a degree that makes the individual dependent on others. Complicated daily tasks or recreational activities cannot be undertaken.

Moderate. The decline in cognitive abilities makes the individual unable to function without the assistance of another in daily living, including shopping and handling money. Within the home, only simple chores can be performed. Activities are increasingly restricted and poorly sustained.

Severe. The decline is characterized by an absence, or virtual absence, of intelligible ideation.

The overall severity of the dementia is best expressed as the level of decline in memory *or* other cognitive abilities, whichever is the more severe (e.g. mild decline in memory *and* moderate decline in cognitive abilities indicate a dementia of moderate severity).

G2. Awareness of the environment (i.e. absence of clouding of consciousness (as defined in F05.–, criterion A)) is preserved during a period of time sufficiently long to allow the unequivocal demonstration of the symptoms in criterion G1. When there are superimposed episodes of delirium, the diagnosis of dementia should be deferred.

G3. There is a decline in emotional control or motivation, or a change in social behaviour manifest as at least one of the following:

(1) emotional lability;

(2) irritability;

(3) apathy;

(4) coarsening of social behaviour.

G4. For a confident clinical diagnosis, the symptoms in criterion G1 should have been present for at least 6 months; if the period since the manifest onset is shorter, the diagnosis can be only tentative.

Comments

The diagnosis is further supported by evidence of damage to other higher cortical functions, such as aphasia, agnosia, apraxia.

Judgement about independent living or the development of dependence (upon others) should take account of the cultural expectation and context.

Dementia is specified here as having a minimum duration of 6 months to avoid confusion with reversible states with identical behavioural syndromes, such as traumatic subdural haemorrhage (S06.5), normal pressure hydrocephalus (G91.2) and diffuse or focal brain injury (S06.2 and S06.3).

A fifth character may be used to indicate the presence of additional symptoms in the categories F00–F03 (F00.– Dementia in Alzheimer's disease; F01.– Vascular dementia; F02.– Dementia in diseases classified elsewhere; F03.– Unspecified dementia), as follows:

.*x*0 Without additional symptoms
.*x*1 With other symptoms, predominantly delusional
.*x*2 With other symptoms, predominantly hallucinatory
.*x*3 With other symptoms, predominantly depressive
.*x*4 With other mixed symptoms

A sixth character may be used to indicate the severity of the dementia:

.*xx*0 Mild
.*xx*1 Moderate
.*xx*2 Severe

As mentioned above on page 30, the overall severity of the dementia depends on the level of memory *or* intellectual impairment, whichever is the more severe.

F00 Dementia in Alzheimer's disease

A. The general criteria for dementia G1–G4 must be met.

B. There is no evidence from the history, physical examination, or special investigations for any other possible cause of dementia (e.g. cerebrovascular disease, HIV disease, Parkinson's disease, Huntington's disease, normal pressure hydrocephalus), a systemic disorder (e.g. hypothyroidism, vitamin B_{12} or folic acid deficiency, hypercalcaemia), or alcohol or drug abuse.

Comments

The diagnosis is confirmed by post-mortem evidence of neurofibrillary tangles and neuritic plaques in excess of those found in normal aging of the brain.

The following features support the diagnosis, but are not necessary elements: involvement of cortical functions as evidenced by aphasia, agnosia or apraxia; decrease of motivation and drive, leading to apathy and lack of spontaneity; irritability and disinhibition of social behaviour; evidence from special investigations that there is cerebral atrophy, particularly if this can be shown to be increasing over time. In severe cases there may be Parkinson-like extrapyramidal changes, logoclonia, and epileptic fits.

Specification of features for possible subtypes

Because of the possibility that subtypes exist, it is recommended that the following characteristics be ascertained as a basis for a further classification: age at onset; rate of progression; configuration of the clinical features, particularly the relative prominence (or lack) of temporal, parietal, or frontal lobe signs; any neuropathological or neurochemical abnormalities, and their pattern.

The division of Alzheimer's disease into subtypes can at present be accomplished in two ways: first by taking only the age of onset and labelling the disease as either early or late, with an approximate cut-off point at 65 years; or second, by assessing how well the individual conforms to one of the two putative syndromes, early- or late-onset type.

It should be noted that a sharp distinction between early- and late-onset types is unlikely. Early-onset type may occur in late life, just as late-onset type may occasionally have an onset before the age of 65. The following criteria may be used to differentiate F00.0 from F00.1, but it should be remembered that the status of this subdivision is still controversial.

F00.0 Dementia in Alzheimer's disease with early onset

1. The criteria for dementia in Alzheimer's disease (F00) must be met, and the age at onset must be below 65 years.

2. In addition, at least one of the following requirements must be met:

(a) evidence of a relatively rapid onset and progression;
(b) in addition to memory impairment, there must be aphasia (amnesic or sensory), agraphia, alexia, acalculia, or apraxia (indicating the presence of temporal, parietal, and/or frontal lobe involvement).

F00.1 Dementia in Alzheimer's disease with late onset

1. The criteria for dementia in Alzheimer's disease (F00) must be met and the age at onset must be 65 years or more.

2. In addition, at least one of the following requirements must be met:
   (a) evidence of a very slow, gradual onset and progression (the rate of the latter may be known only retrospectively after a course of 3 years or more);
   (b) predominance of memory impairment G1(1), over intellectual impairment G1(2) (see general criteria for dementia).

F00.2 Dementia in Alzheimer's disease, atypical or mixed type

This term and code should be used for dementias that have important atypical features or that fulfil criteria for both early- and late-onset types of Alzheimer's disease. Mixed Alzheimer's and vascular dementia is also included here.

F00.9 Dementia in Alzheimer's disease, unspecified

F01 Vascular dementia

G1. The general criteria for dementia (G1–G4) must be met.

G2. Deficits in higher cognitive functions are unevenly distributed, with some functions affected and others relatively spared. Thus memory may be quite markedly affected while thinking, reasoning, and information processing may show only mild decline.

G3. There is clinical evidence of focal brain damage, manifest as at least one of the following:

(1) unilateral spastic weakness of the limbs;
(2) unilaterally increased tendon reflexes;
(3) an extensor plantar response;
(4) pseudobulbar palsy.

G4. There is evidence from the history, examination, or tests of a significant cerebrovascular disease, which may reasonably be judged to be etiologically related to the dementia (e.g. a history of stroke; evidence of cerebral infarction).

The following criteria may be used to differentiate subtypes of vascular dementia, but it should be remembered that the usefulness of this subdivision may not be generally accepted.

F01.0 Vascular dementia of acute onset

A. The general criteria for vascular dementia (F01) must be met.

B. The dementia develops rapidly (i.e. usually within 1 month, but within no longer than 3 months) after a succession of strokes or (rarely) after a single large infarction.

F01.1 Multi-infarct dementia

A. The general criteria for vascular dementia (F01) must be met.

B. The onset of the dementia is gradual (i.e. within 3–6 months), following a number of minor ischaemic episodes.

Comments

It is presumed that there is an accumulation of infarcts in the cerebral parenchyma. Between the ischaemic episodes there may be periods of actual clinical improvement.

F01.2 Subcortical vascular dementia

A. The general criteria for vascular dementia (F01) must be met.

B. There is a history of hypertension.

C. There is evidence from clinical examination and special investigations of vascular disease located in the deep white matter of the cerebral hemispheres, with preservation of the cerebral cortex.

F01.3 Mixed cortical and subcortical vascular dementia

Mixed cortical and subcortical components of the vascular dementia may be suspected from the clinical features, the results of investigations (including autopsy) or both.

F01.8 Other vascular dementia

F01.9 Vascular dementia, unspecified

F02 Dementia in other diseases classified elsewhere

F02.0 Dementia in Pick's disease

A. The general criteria for dementia (G1–G4) must be met.

B. Onset is slow with steady deterioration.

C. Predominance of frontal lobe involvement is evidenced by two or more of the following:

(1) emotional blunting;
(2) coarsening of social behaviour;
(3) disinhibition;
(4) apathy or restlessness;
(5) aphasia.

D. In the early stages, memory and parietal lobe functions are relatively preserved.

F02.1 Dementia in Creutzfeldt–Jakob disease

A. The general criteria for dementia (G1–G4) must be met.

B. There is very rapid progression of the dementia, with disintegration of virtually all higher cerebral functions.

C. One or more of the following types of neurological symptoms and signs emerge, usually after or simultaneously with the dementia:

(1) pyramidal symptoms;
(2) extrapyramidal symptoms;
(3) cerebellar symptoms;
(4) aphasia;
(5) visual impairment.

Comments

An akinetic and mute state is the typical terminal stage. An amyotrophic variant may be seen, where the neurological signs precede the onset of the dementia. A characteristic electroencephalogram (periodic spikes against a slow and low voltage background), if present in association with the above clinical signs, will increase the probability of the diagnosis. However, the diagnosis can be confirmed only by neuropathological examination (neuronal loss, astrocytosis, and spongiform changes). Because of the risk of infection, this should be carried out only under special protective conditions.

F02.2 Dementia in Huntington's disease

A. The general criteria for dementia (G1–G4) must be met.

B. Subcortical functions are affected first and dominate the picture of dementia throughout; subcortical involvement is manifested by slowness of thinking or movement and personality alteration with apathy or depression.

C. There are involuntary choreiform movements, typically of the face, hands, or shoulders, or in the gait. The patient may attempt to conceal them by converting them into a voluntary action.

D. There is a history of Huntington's disease in one parent or a sibling, or a family history that suggests the disorder.

E. There are no clinical features that otherwise account for the abnormal movements.

Comments

In addition to involuntary choreiform movements, there may be development of extrapyramidal rigidity or of spasticity with pyramidal signs.

F02.3 Dementia in Parkinson's disease

A. The general criteria for dementia (G1–G4) must be met.

B. A diagnosis of Parkinson's disease has been established.

C. None of the cognitive impairment is attributable to anti-parkinsonian medication.

D. There is no evidence from the history, physical examination, or special investigations for any other possible cause of dementia, including other forms of brain disease, damage, or dysfunction (e.g. cerebrovascular disease, HIV disease, Huntington's disease, normal pressure hydrocephalus), a systemic disorder (e.g. hypothyroidism, vitamin B_{12} or folic acid deficiency, hypercalcaemia), or alcohol or drug abuse.

If criteria are also fulfilled for dementia in Alzheimer's disease with late onset (F00.1), category F00.1 should be used in combination with G20 (Parkinson's disease).

F02.4 Dementia in human immunodeficiency virus [HIV] disease

A. The general criteria for dementia (G1–G4) must be met.

B. A diagnosis of HIV infection has been established.

C. There is no evidence from the history, physical examination, or special investigations for any other possible cause of dementia, including other forms of brain disease, damage, or dysfunction (e.g. Alzheimer's disease, cerebrovascular disease, Parkinson's disease, Huntington's disease, normal pressure hydrocephalus), a systemic disorder (e.g. hypothyroidism, vitamin B_{12} or folic acid deficiency, hypercalcaemia), or alcohol or drug abuse.

F02.8 Dementia in other specified diseases classified elsewhere

Dementia can occur as a manifestation or consequence of a variety of cerebral and somatic conditions. To specify the etiology, the ICD-10 code for the underlying condition should be added.

F03 Unspecified dementia

This category should be used when the general criteria for dementia are met, but when it is not possible to identify one of the specific types (F00.0–F02.9).

F04 Organic amnesic syndrome, not induced by alcohol and other psychoactive substances

A. There is memory impairment, manifest in both:
   (1) a defect of recent memory (impaired learning of new material), to a degree sufficient to interfere with daily living; and
   (2) a reduced ability to recall past experiences.

B. There is no:
   (1) defect in immediate recall (as tested, for example, by the digit span);
   (2) clouding of consciousness and disturbance of attention, as defined in F05.–, criterion A;
   (3) global intellectual decline (dementia).

C. There is objective evidence (from physical and neurological examination, laboratory tests) and/or history of an insult to, or a disease of, the brain (especially involving bilaterally the diencephalic and medial temporal structures but other than alcoholic encephalopathy) that can reasonably be presumed to be responsible for the clinical manifestations described in criterion A.

Comments

Associated features, including confabulations, emotional changes (apathy, lack of initiative), and lack of insight are useful additional pointers to the diagnosis but are not invariably present.

F05 Delirium, not induced by alcohol and other psychoactive substances

A. There is clouding of consciousness, i.e. reduced clarity of awareness of the environment, with reduced ability to focus, sustain, or shift attention.

B. Disturbance of cognition is manifest by both:
   (1) impairment of immediate recall and recent memory, with relatively intact remote memory;
   (2) disorientation in time, place or person.

C. At least one of the following psychomotor disturbances is present:
   (1) rapid, unpredictable shifts from hypoactivity to hyperactivity;
   (2) increased reaction time;
   (3) increased or decreased flow of speech;
   (4) enhanced startle reaction.

D. There is disturbance of sleep or of the sleep–wake cycle, manifest by at least one of the following:

(1) insomnia, which in severe cases may involve total sleep loss, with or without daytime drowsiness, or reversal of the sleep–wake cycle;
(2) nocturnal worsening of symptoms;
(3) disturbing dreams and nightmares, which may continue as hallucinations or illusions after awakening.

E. Symptoms have rapid onset and show fluctuations over the course of the day.

F. There is objective evidence from history, physical and neurological examination, or laboratory tests of an underlying cerebral or systemic disease (other than psychoactive substance-related) that can be presumed to be responsible for the clinical manifestations in criteria A–D.

Comments

Emotional disturbances such as depression, anxiety or fear, irritability, euphoria, apathy, or wondering perplexity, disturbances of perception (illusions or hallucinations, often visual), and transient delusions are typical but are not specific indications for the diagnosis.

A fourth character may be used to indicate whether or not the delirium is superimposed on dementia:

F05.0 Delirium, not superimposed on dementia

F05.1 Delirium, superimposed on dementia

F05.8 Other delirium

F05.9 Delirium, unspecified

F06 Other mental disorders due to brain damage and dysfunction and to physical disease

G1. There is objective evidence (from physical and neurological examination and laboratory tests) and/or history of cerebral disease, damage, or dysfunction, or of systemic physical disorder known to cause cerebral dysfunction, including hormonal disturbances (other than alcohol- or other psychoactive substance-related) and non-psychoactive drug effects.

G2. There is a presumed relationship between the development (or marked exacerbation) of the underlying disease, damage, or dysfunction, and the mental disorder, the symptoms of which may have immediate onset or may be delayed.

G3. There is recovery from or significant improvement in the mental disorder following removal or improvement of the underlying presumed cause.

G4. There is insufficient evidence for an alternative causation of the mental disorder, e.g. a strong family history of a clinically similar or related disorder.

If criteria G1, G2, and G4 are met, a provisional diagnosis is justified; if, in addition, there is evidence of G3, the diagnosis can be regarded as certain.

F06.0 Organic hallucinosis

A. The general criteria for F06 must be met.

B. The clinical picture is dominated by persistent or recurrent hallucinations (usually visual or auditory).

C. Hallucinations occur in clear consciousness.

Comments

Delusional elaboration of the hallucinations, as well as full or partial insight, may or may not be present: these features are not essential for the diagnosis.

F06.1 Organic catatonic disorder

A. The general criteria for F06 must be met.

B. One of the following must be present:

(1) stupor, i.e. profound diminution or absence of voluntary movements and speech, and of normal responsiveness to light, noise, and touch, but with normal muscle tone, static posture, and breathing maintained (and often limited coordinated eye movements);

(2) negativism (positive resistance to passive movement of limbs or body or rigid posturing).

C. There is catatonic excitement (gross hypermotility of a chaotic quality, with or without a tendency to assaultiveness).

D. There is rapid and unpredictable alternation of stupor and excitement.

Comments

Confidence in the diagnosis will be increased if additional catatonic phenomena are present, e.g. stereotypies, waxy flexibility, and impulsive acts. Care should be taken to exclude delirium; however, it is not known at present whether an organic catatonic state always occurs in clear consciousness, or whether it represents an atypical manifestation of a delirium in which criteria A, B, and D are only marginally met while criterion C is prominent.

F06.2 Organic delusional [schizophrenia-like] disorder

A. The general criteria for F06 must be met.

B. The clinical picture is dominated by delusions (of persecution, bodily change, disease, death, jealousy), which may exhibit a varying degree of systematization.

C. Consciousness is clear and memory is intact.

Comments

Further features that complete the clinical picture but that are not invariably present include: hallucinations (in any modality); schizophrenic-type thought disorder; isolated catatonic phenomena such as stereotypies, negativism, or impulsive acts.

The clinical picture may meet the symptomatic criteria for schizophrenia (F20.0–F20.3), persistent delusional disorder (F22.–), or acute and transient psychotic disorders (F23.–). However, if the state also meets the general criteria for a presumptive organic etiology laid down in the introduction to F06, it should be classified here. It should be noted that marginal or nonspecific findings such as enlarged cerebral ventricles or "soft" neurological signs *do not qualify as evidence* for criterion G1 of F06.

F06.3 Organic mood [affective] disorder

A. The general criteria for F06 must be met.

B. The condition must meet the criteria for one of the affective disorders laid down in F30–F38.

The diagnosis of the affective disorder may be specified by using a fifth character:

F06.30 Organic manic disorder

F06.31 Organic bipolar disorder

F06.32 Organic depressive disorder

F06.33 Organic mixed affective disorder

F06.4 Organic anxiety disorder

A. The general criteria for F06 must be met.

B. The condition must meet the criteria for either F41.0 or F41.1.

F06.5 Organic dissociative disorder

A. The general criteria for F06 must be met.

B. The condition must meet the criteria for one of the categories F44.0–F44.8.

F06.6 Organic emotionally labile [asthenic] disorder

A. The general criteria for F06 must be met.

B. The clinical picture is dominated by emotional lability (uncontrolled, unstable, and fluctuating expression of emotions).

C. There is a variety of unpleasant physical sensations such as dizziness or pains and aches.

Comments

Fatiguability and listlessness (asthenia) are often present but are not essential for the diagnosis.

F06.7 Mild cognitive disorder

Note: The status of this construct is being examined. Specific research criteria must be viewed as tentative. One of the principal reasons for its inclusion is to obtain further evidence allowing its differentiation from disorders such as dementia (F00–F03), organic amnesic syndrome (F04), delirium (F05.–), and several disorders in F07.–.

A. The general criteria for F06 must be met.

B. There is a disorder in cognitive function for most of the time over a period of at least 2 weeks, as reported by the individual or a reliable informant. The disorder is exemplified by difficulties in any of the following areas:
   (1) memory (particularly recall) or new learning;
   (2) attention or concentration;
   (3) thinking (e.g. slowing in problem-solving or abstraction);
   (4) language (e.g. comprehension, word-finding);
   (5) visual-spatial functioning.

C. There is an abnormality or decline in performance in quantified cognitive assessments (e.g. neuropsychological tests or mental status examination).

D. None of the difficulties listed in criterion B (1)–(5) is such that a diagnosis can be made of dementia (F00–F03), organic amnesic syndrome (F04), delirium (F05.–), postencephalitic syndrome (F07.1), postconcussional syndrome (F07.2), or other persisting cognitive impairment due to psychoactive substance use (F1*x*.74).

Comments

If criterion G1 for F06 is fulfilled by the presence of central nervous system dysfunction, it is usually presumed that this is the cause of the mild cognitive disorder. If criterion G1 is fulfilled by the presence of a systemic physical disorder, it is often unjustified to assume that there is a direct causative relationship. Nevertheless, it may be useful in such instances to record the presence of the systemic physical disorder as "associated", without implying a necessary causation. An additional fifth character may be used for this:

F06.70 Not associated with a systemic physical disorder

F06.71 Associated with a systemic physical disorder

The systemic physical disorder should be recorded separately by its appropriate ICD-10 code.

F06.8 Other specified mental disorders due to brain damage and dysfunction and to physical disease

Examples of this category are transient or mild abnormal mood states occurring during treatment with steroids or antidepressants which do not meet the criteria for organic mood disorder (F06.3).

F06.9 Unspecified mental disorder due to brain damage and dysfunction and to physical disease

F07 Personality and behavioural disorders due to brain disease, damage and dysfunction

G1. There must be objective evidence (from physical and neurological examination and laboratory tests) and/or history of cerebral disease, damage, or dysfunction.

G2. There is no clouding of consciousness or significant memory deficit.

G3. There is insufficient evidence for an alternative causation of the personality or behaviour disorder that would justify its placement in F60–F69.

F07.0 Organic personality disorder

A. The general criteria for F07 must be met.

B. At least three of the following features must be present over a period of 6 months or more:

(1) consistently reduced ability to persevere with goal-directed activities, especially those involving relatively long periods of time and postponed gratification;

(2) one or more of the following emotional changes:

(a) emotional lability (uncontrolled, unstable, and fluctuating expression of emotions);
(b) euphoria and shallow, inappropriate jocularity, unwarranted by the circumstances;
(c) irritability and/or outbursts of anger and aggression;
(d) apathy;

(3) disinhibited expression of needs or impulses without consideration of consequences or of social conventions (the indi-

vidual may engage in dissocial acts such as stealing, inappropriate sexual advances, or voracious eating, or exhibit extreme disregard for personal hygiene);

(4) cognitive disturbances, typically in the form of:

(a) excessive suspiciousness and paranoid ideas;

(b) excessive preoccupation with a single theme such as religion, or rigid categorization of other people's behaviour in terms of "right" and "wrong";

(5) marked alteration of the rate and flow of language production, with features such as circumstantiality, over-inclusiveness, viscosity, and hypergraphia;

(6) altered sexual behaviour (hyposexuality or change in sexual preference).

Specification of features for possible subtypes

Option 1. A marked predominance of the symptoms in criteria (1) and (2)(d) is thought to define a pseudoretarded or apathetic type, a predominance of (1), (2)(c), and (3) is considered a pseudopsychopathic type; and a combination of (4), (5) and (6) is regarded as characteristic of the limbic epilepsy personality syndrome. None of these entities has yet been sufficiently validated to warrant a separate description.

Option 2. If desired, the following types may be specified: labile type, disinhibited type, aggressive type, apathetic type, paranoid type, mixed type, and other.

F07.1 Postencephalitic syndrome

A. The general criteria for F07 must be met.

B. At least one of the following residual neurological dysfunctions must be present:

(1) paralysis;
(2) deafness;
(3) aphasia;
(4) constructional apraxia;
(5) acalculia.

C. The syndrome is reversible, and its duration rarely exceeds 24 months.

Comments

Criterion C constitutes the main difference between this disorder and organic personality disorder (F07.0).

Residual symptoms and behavioural change following either viral or bacterial encephalitis are nonspecific and do not provide a sufficient basis for a clinical diagnosis. They may include: general malaise, apathy, or irritability; some lowering of cognitive functioning (learning difficulties); disturbances in the sleep–wake pattern; or altered sexual behaviour.

F07.2 Postconcussional syndrome

Note. The nosological status of this syndrome is uncertain, and criterion G1 of the introduction to this rubric is not always ascertainable. However, for those undertaking research into this condition, the following criteria are recommended:

A. The general criteria of F07 must be met.

B. There must be a history of head trauma with loss of consciousness, preceding the onset of symptoms by a period of up to 4 weeks. (Objective EEG, brain imaging, or oculonystagmographic evidence for brain damage may be lacking.)

C. At least three of the following features must be present:

(1) complaints of unpleasant sensations and pains, such as headache, dizziness (usually lacking the features of true vertigo), general malaise and excessive fatigue, or noise intolerance;

(2) emotional changes, such as irritability, emotional lability (both easily provoked or exacerbated by emotional excitement or stress), or some degree of depression and/or anxiety;

(3) subjective complaints of difficulty in concentration and in performing mental tasks, and of memory problems (without clear objective evidence, e.g. psychological tests, of marked impairment);

(4) insomnia;

(5) reduced tolerance to alcohol;

(6) preoccupation with the above symptoms and fear of permanent brain damage, to the extent of hypochondriacal, overvalued ideas and adoption of a sick role.

F07.8 Other organic personality and behavioural disorders due to brain disease, damage and dysfunction

Brain disease, damage, or dysfunction may produce a variety of cognitive, emotional, personality, and behavioural disorders, some of which may not be classifiable under F07.0–F07.2. However, since the nosological status of the tentative syndromes in this area is uncertain, they should be coded as "other". A fifth character may be added, if necessary, to identify presumptive individual entities.

F07.9 Unspecified organic personality and behavioural disorder due to brain disease, damage and dysfunction

F09 Unspecified organic or symptomatic mental disorder

F10–F19 Mental and behavioural disorders due to psychoactive substance use

F10.– Mental and behavioural disorders due to use of alcohol

F11.– Mental and behavioural disorders due to use of opioids

F12.– Mental and behavioural disorders due to use of cannabinoids

F13.– Mental and behavioural disorders due to use of sedatives or hypnotics

F14.– Mental and behavioural disorders due to use of cocaine

F15.– Mental and behavioural disorders due to use of other stimulants, including caffeine

F16.– Mental and behavioural disorders due to use of hallucinogens

F17.– Mental and behavioural disorders due to use of tobacco

F18.– Mental and behavioural disorders due to use of volatile solvents

F19.– Mental and behavioural disorders due to multiple drug use and use of other psychoactive substances

F1*x*.0 Acute intoxication

G1. There must be clear evidence of recent use of a psychoactive substance (or substances) at sufficiently high dose levels to be consistent with intoxication.

G2. There must be symptoms or signs of intoxication compatible with the known actions of the particular substance (or substances), as specified below, and of sufficient severity to produce disturbances in the level of consciousness, cognition, perception, affect, or behaviour that are of clinical importance.

G3. The symptoms or signs present cannot be accounted for by a medical disorder unrelated to substance use, and not better accounted for by another mental or behavioural disorder.

Acute intoxication frequently occurs in persons who have more persistent alcohol- or drug-related problems in addition. Where there are such problems, e.g. harmful use (F1*x*.1), dependence syndrome (F1*x*.2), or psychotic disorder (F1*x*.5), they should also be recorded.

The following five-character codes may be used to indicate whether the acute intoxication was associated with any complications:

F1*x*.00 Uncomplicated
Symptoms of varying severity, usually dose-dependent.

F1*x*.01 With trauma or other bodily injury

F1*x*.02 With other medical complications
Examples are haematemesis, inhalation of vomit.

F1*x*.03 With delirium

F1*x*.04 With perceptual distortions

F1*x*.05 With coma

F1*x*.06 With convulsions

F1*x*.07 Pathological intoxication
Applies only to alcohol.

F10.0 Acute intoxication due to use of alcohol

A. The general criteria for acute intoxication (F1*x*.0) must be met.

B. There must be dysfunctional behaviour, as evidenced by at least one of the following:

(1) disinhibition;
(2) argumentativeness;
(3) aggression;

(4) lability of mood;
(5) impaired attention;
(6) impaired judgement;
(7) interference with personal functioning.

C. At least one of the following signs must be present:

(1) unsteady gait;
(2) difficulty in standing;
(3) slurred speech;
(4) nystagmus;
(5) decreased level of consciousness (e.g. sopor, coma);
(6) flushed face;
(7) conjunctival injection.

Comment

When severe, acute alcohol intoxication may be accompanied by hypotension, hypothermia, and depression of the gag reflex.

If desired, the blood alcohol level may be specified by using ICD-10 codes Y90.0–Y90.8. Code Y91.– may be used to specify the clinical severity of intoxication if the blood alcohol level is not available.

F10.07 Pathological alcohol intoxication

Note. The status of this condition is being examined. These research criteria must be regarded as tentative.

A. The general criteria for acute intoxication (F1*x*.0) must be met, with the exception that pathological intoxication occurs after drinking amounts of alcohol insufficient to cause intoxication in most people.

B. There is verbally aggressive or physically violent behaviour that is not typical of the person when sober.

C. The intoxication occurs very soon (usually a few minutes) after consumption of alcohol.

D. There is no evidence of organic cerebral disorder or other mental disorders.

Comment

This is an uncommon condition. The blood alcohol levels found in this disorder are lower than those that would cause acute intoxication in most people, i.e. below 40 mg/100 ml.

F11.0 Acute intoxication due to use of opioids

A. The general criteria for acute intoxication (F1*x*.0) must be met.

B. There must be dysfunctional behaviour, as evidenced by at least one of the following:

(1) apathy and sedation;
(2) disinhibition;
(3) psychomotor retardation;
(4) impaired attention;
(5) impaired judgement;
(6) interference with personal functioning.

C. At least one of the following signs must be present:

(1) drowsiness;
(2) slurred speech;
(3) pupillary constriction (except in anoxia from severe overdose, when pupillary dilatation occurs);
(4) decreased level of consciousness (e.g. sopor, coma).

Comment

When severe, acute opioid intoxication may be accompanied by respiratory depression (and hypoxia), hypotension, and hypothermia.

F12.0 Acute intoxication due to use of cannabinoids

A. The general criteria for acute intoxication (F1*x*.0) must be met.

B. There must be dysfunctional behaviour or perceptual abnormalities, including at least one of the following:

(1) euphoria and disinhibition;
(2) anxiety or agitation;
(3) suspiciousness or paranoid ideation;
(4) temporal slowing (a sense that time is passing very slowly, and/or the person is experiencing a rapid flow of ideas);
(5) impaired judgement;

(6) impaired attention;
(7) impaired reaction time;
(8) auditory, visual, or tactile illusions;
(9) hallucinations with preserved orientation;
(10) depersonalization;
(11) derealization;
(12) interference with personal functioning.

C. At least one of the following signs must be present:

(1) increased appetite;
(2) dry mouth;
(3) conjunctival injection;
(4) tachycardia.

F13.0 Acute intoxication due to use of sedatives or hypnotics

A. The general criteria for acute intoxication (F1*x*.0) must be met.

B. There is dysfunctional behaviour, as evidenced by at least one of the following:

(1) euphoria and disinhibition;
(2) apathy and sedation;
(3) abusiveness or aggression;
(4) lability of mood;
(5) impaired attention;
(6) anterograde amnesia;
(7) impaired psychomotor performance;
(8) interference with personal functioning.

C. At least one of the following signs must be present:

(1) unsteady gait;
(2) difficulty in standing;
(3) slurred speech;
(4) nystagmus;
(5) decreased level of consciousness (e.g. sopor, coma);
(6) erythematous skin lesions or blisters.

Comment

When severe, acute intoxication from sedative or hypnotic drugs may be accompanied by hypotension, hypothermia, and depression of the gag reflex.

F14.0 Acute intoxication due to use of cocaine

A. The general criteria for acute intoxication (F1*x*.0) must be met.

B. There must be dysfunctional behaviour or perceptual abnormalities, as evidenced by at least one of the following:

(1) euphoria and sensation of increased energy;
(2) hypervigilance;
(3) grandiose beliefs or actions;
(4) abusiveness or aggression;
(5) argumentativeness;
(6) lability of mood;
(7) repetitive stereotyped behaviours;
(8) auditory, visual, or tactile illusions;
(9) hallucinations, usually with intact orientation;
(10) paranoid ideation;
(11) interference with personal functioning.

C. At least two of the following signs must be present:

(1) tachycardia (sometimes bradycardia);
(2) cardiac arrhythmias;
(3) hypertension (sometimes hypotension);
(4) sweating and chills;
(5) nausea or vomiting;
(6) evidence of weight loss;
(7) pupillary dilatation;
(8) psychomotor agitation (sometimes retardation);
(9) muscular weakness;
(10) chest pain;
(11) convulsions.

Comment

Interference with personal functioning is most readily apparent from the social interactions of cocaine users, which range from extreme gregariousness to social withdrawal.

F15.0 Acute intoxication due to use of other stimulants, including caffeine

A. The general criteria for acute intoxication (F1*x*.0) must be met.

B. There must be dysfunctional behaviour or perceptual abnormalities, as evidenced by at least one of the following:

(1) euphoria and sensation of increased energy;
(2) hypervigilance;
(3) grandiose beliefs or actions;
(4) abusiveness or aggression;
(5) argumentativeness;
(6) lability of mood;
(7) repetitive stereotyped behaviours;
(8) auditory, visual, or tactile illusions;
(9) hallucinations, usually with intact orientation;
(10) paranoid ideation;
(11) interference with personal functioning.

C. At least two of the following signs must be present:

(1) tachycardia (sometimes bradycardia);
(2) cardiac arrhythmias;
(3) hypertension (sometimes hypotension);
(4) sweating and chills;
(5) nausea or vomiting;
(6) evidence of weight loss;
(7) pupillary dilatation;
(8) psychomotor agitation (sometimes retardation);
(9) muscular weakness;
(10) chest pain;
(11) convulsions.

Comment

Interference with personal functioning is most readily apparent from the social interactions of the substance users, which range from extreme gregariousness to social withdrawal.

F16.0 Acute intoxication due to use of hallucinogens

A. The general criteria for acute intoxication (F1*x*.0) must be met.

B. There must be dysfunctional behaviour or perceptual abnormalities, as evidenced by at least one of the following:

(1) anxiety and fearfulness;
(2) auditory, visual, or tactile illusions or hallucinations occurring in a state of full wakefulness and alertness;
(3) depersonalization;
(4) derealization;
(5) paranoid ideation;

(6) ideas of reference;
(7) lability of mood;
(8) hyperactivity;
(9) impulsive acts;
(10) impaired attention;
(11) interference with personal functioning.

C. At least two of the following signs must be present:

(1) tachycardia;
(2) palpitations;
(3) sweating and chills;
(4) tremor;
(5) blurring of vision;
(6) pupillary dilatation;
(7) incoordination.

F17.0 Acute intoxication due to use of tobacco [acute nicotine intoxication]

A. The general criteria for acute intoxication (F1*x*.0) must be met.

B. There must be dysfunctional behaviour or perceptual abnormalities, as evidenced by at least one of the following:

(1) insomnia;
(2) bizarre dreams;
(3) lability of mood;
(4) derealization;
(5) interference with personal functioning.

C. At least one of the following signs must be present:

(1) nausea or vomiting;
(2) sweating;
(3) tachycardia;
(4) cardiac arrhythmias.

F18.0 Acute intoxication due to use of volatile solvents

A. The general criteria for acute intoxication (F1*x*.0) must be met.

B. There must be dysfunctional behaviour, evidenced by at least one of the following:

(1) apathy and lethargy;
(2) argumentativeness;

(3) abusiveness or aggression;
(4) lability of mood;
(5) impaired judgement;
(6) impaired attention and memory;
(7) psychomotor retardation;
(8) interference with personal functioning.

C. At least one of the following signs must be present:

(1) unsteady gait;
(2) difficulty in standing;
(3) slurred speech;
(4) nystagmus;
(5) decreased level of consciousness (e.g. sopor, coma);
(6) muscle weakness;
(7) blurred vision or diplopia.

Comment

Acute intoxication from inhalation of substances other than solvents should also be coded here.

When severe, acute intoxication from volatile solvents may be accompanied by hypotension, hypothermia, and depression of the gag reflex.

F19.0 Acute intoxication due to multiple drug use and use of other psychoactive substances

This category should be used when there is evidence of intoxication caused by recent use of other psychoactive substances (e.g. phencyclidine) or of multiple psychoactive substances where it is uncertain which substance has predominated.

F1*x*.1 Harmful use

A. There must be clear evidence that the substance use was responsible for (or substantially contributed to) physical or psychological harm, including impaired judgement or dysfunctional behaviour, which may lead to disability or have adverse consequences for interpersonal relationships.

B. The nature of the harm should be clearly identifiable (and specified).

C. The pattern of use has persisted for at least 1 month or has occurred repeatedly within a 12-month period.

D. The disorder does not meet the criteria for any other mental or behavioural disorder related to the same drug in the same time period (except for acute intoxication, F1*x*.0).

F1*x*.2 Dependence syndrome

A. Three or more of the following manifestations should have occurred together for at least 1 month or, if persisting for periods of less than 1 month, should have occurred together repeatedly within a 12-month period:

(1) a strong desire or sense of compulsion to take the substance;

(2) impaired capacity to control substance-taking behaviour in terms of its onset, termination, or levels of use, as evidenced by: the substance being often taken in larger amounts or over a longer period than intended; or by a persistent desire or unsuccessful efforts to reduce or control substance use;

(3) a physiological withdrawal state (see F1*x*.3 and F1*x*.4) when substance use is reduced or ceased, as evidenced by the characteristic withdrawal syndrome for the substance, or by use of the same (or closely related) substance with the intention of relieving or avoiding withdrawal symptoms;

(4) evidence of tolerance to the effects of the substance, such that there is a need for significantly increased amounts of the substance to achieve intoxication or the desired effect, or a markedly diminished effect with continued use of the same amount of the substance;

(5) preoccupation with substance use, as manifested by important alternative pleasures or interests being given up or reduced because of substance use; or a great deal of time being spent in activities necessary to obtain, take, or recover from the effects of the substance;

(6) persistent substance use despite clear evidence of harmful consequences (see F1*x*.1), as evidenced by continued use when the individual is actually aware, or may be expected to be aware, of the nature and extent of harm.

Diagnosis of the dependence syndrome may be further specified by the following five- and six-character codes:

F1*x*.20 Currently abstinent
- F1*x*.200 Early remission
- F1*x*.201 Partial remission
- F1*x*.202 Full remission

F1*x*.21 Currently abstinent but in a protected environment
(e.g. in hospital, in a therapeutic community, in prison, etc.)

F1*x*.22 Currently on a clinically supervised maintenance or replacement regime [controlled dependence]
(e.g. with methadone; nicotine gum or nicotine patch)

F1*x*.23 Currently abstinent, but receiving treatment with aversive or blocking drugs
(e.g. naltrexone or disulfiram)

F1*x*.24 Currently using the substance [active dependence]
- F1*x*.240 Without physical features
- F1*x*.241 With physical features

The course of the dependence may be further specified, if desired, as follows:

F1*x*.25 Continuous use

F1*x*.26 Episodic use [dipsomania]

F1*x*.3 Withdrawal state

G1. There must be clear evidence of recent cessation or reduction of substance use after repeated, and usually prolonged and/or high-dose, use of that substance.

G2. Symptoms and signs are compatible with the known features of a withdrawal state from the particular substance or substances (see below).

G3. Symptoms and signs are not accounted for by a medical disorder unrelated to substance use, and not better accounted for by another mental or behavioural disorder.

The diagnosis of withdrawal state may be further specified by using the following five-character codes:

F1*x*.30 Uncomplicated

F1*x*.31 With convulsions

F10.3 Alcohol withdrawal state

A. The general criteria for withdrawal state (F1*x*.3) must be met.

B. Any three of the following signs must be present:

(1) tremor of the tongue, eyelids, or outstretched hands;
(2) sweating;
(3) nausea, retching, or vomiting;
(4) tachycardia or hypertension;
(5) psychomotor agitation;
(6) headache;
(7) insomnia;
(8) malaise or weakness;
(9) transient visual, tactile, or auditory hallucinations or illusions;
(10) grand mal convulsions.

Comment

If delirium is present, the diagnosis should be alcohol withdrawal state with delirium (delirium tremens) (F10.4).

F11.3 Opioid withdrawal state

A. The general criteria for withdrawal state (F1*x*.3) must be met. (Note that an opioid withdrawal state may also be induced by administration of an opioid antagonist after a brief period of opioid use.)

B. Any three of the following signs must be present:

(1) craving for an opioid drug;
(2) rhinorrhoea or sneezing;
(3) lacrimation;
(4) muscle aches or cramps;
(5) abdominal cramps;
(6) nausea or vomiting;
(7) diarrhoea;
(8) pupillary dilatation;
(9) piloerection, or recurrent chills;
(10) tachycardia or hypertension;
(11) yawning;
(12) restless sleep.

F12.3 Cannabinoid withdrawal state

Note. This is an ill-defined syndrome for which definitive diagnostic criteria cannot be established at the present time. It occurs following cessation of prolonged high-dose use of cannabis. It has been reported variously as lasting from several hours to up to 7 days.

Symptoms and signs include anxiety, irritability, tremor of the outstretched hands, sweating, and muscle aches.

F13.3 Sedative or hypnotic withdrawal state

A. The general criteria for withdrawal state (F1*x*.3) must be met.

B. Any three of the following signs must be present:

(1) tremor of the tongue, eyelids, or outstretched hands;
(2) nausea or vomiting;
(3) tachycardia;
(4) postural hypotension;
(5) psychomotor agitation;
(6) headache;
(7) insomnia;
(8) malaise or weakness;
(9) transient visual, tactile, or auditory hallucinations or illusions;
(10) paranoid ideation;
(11) grand mal convulsions.

Comment

If delirium is present, the diagnosis should be sedative or hypnotic withdrawal state with delirium (F13.4).

F14.3 Cocaine withdrawal state

A. The general criteria for withdrawal state (F1*x*.3) must be met.

B. There is dysphoric mood (for instance, sadness or anhedonia).

C. Any two of the following signs must be present:

(1) lethargy and fatigue;
(2) psychomotor retardation or agitation;
(3) craving for cocaine;
(4) increased appetite;
(5) insomnia or hypersomnia;
(6) bizarre or unpleasant dreams.

F15.3 Withdrawal state from other stimulants, including caffeine

A. The general criteria for withdrawal state (F1*x*.3) must be met.

B. There is dysphoric mood (for instance, sadness or anhedonia).

C. Any two of the following signs must be present:

(1) lethargy and fatigue;
(2) psychomotor retardation or agitation;
(3) craving for stimulant drugs;
(4) increased appetite;
(5) insomnia or hypersomnia;
(6) bizarre or unpleasant dreams.

F16.3 Hallucinogen withdrawal state

Note: There is no recognized hallucinogen withdrawal state.

F17.3 Tobacco withdrawal state

A. The general criteria for withdrawal state (F1*x*.3) must be met.

B. Any two of the following signs must be present:

(1) craving for tobacco (or other nicotine-containing products);
(2) malaise or weakness;
(3) anxiety;
(4) dysphoric mood;
(5) irritability or restlessness;
(6) insomnia;
(7) increased appetite;
(8) increased cough;
(9) mouth ulceration;
(10) difficulty in concentrating.

F18.3 Volatile solvents withdrawal state

Note: There is inadequate information on withdrawal states from volatile solvents for research criteria to be formulated.

F19.3 Multiple drugs withdrawal state

F1*x*.4 Withdrawal state with delirium

A. The general criteria for withdrawal state (F1*x*.3) must be met.

B. The criteria for delirium (F05.–) must be met.

The diagnosis of withdrawal state with delirium may be further specified by using the following five-character codes:

F1*x*.40 Without convulsions

F1*x*.41 With convulsions

F1*x*.5 Psychotic disorder

A. Onset of psychotic symptoms must occur during or within 2 weeks of substance use.

B. The psychotic symptoms must persist for more than 48 hours.

C. Duration of the disorder must not exceed 6 months.

The diagnosis of psychotic disorder may be further specified by using the following five-character codes:

F1*x*.50 Schizophrenia-like

F1*x*.51 Predominantly delusional

F1*x*.52 Predominantly hallucinatory

F1*x*.53 Predominantly polymorphic

F1*x*.54 Predominantly depressive symptoms

F1*x*.55 Predominantly manic symptoms

F1*x*.56 Mixed

For research purposes it is recommended that change of the disorder from a non-psychotic to a clearly psychotic state be further specified as either abrupt (onset within 48 hours) or acute (onset in more than 48 hours but less than 2 weeks).

F1*x*.6 Amnesic syndrome

A. Memory impairment is manifest in both:

(1) a defect of recent memory (impaired learning of new material) to a degree sufficient to interfere with daily living; and

(2) a reduced ability to recall past experiences.

B. All of the following are absent (or relatively absent):

(1) defect in immediate recall (as tested, for example, by the digit span);

(2) clouding of consciousness and disturbance of attention, as defined in F05.–, criterion A;

(3) global intellectual decline (dementia).

C. There is no objective evidence from physical and neurological examination, laboratory tests, or history of a disorder or disease of the brain (especially involving bilaterally the diencephalic and medial temporal structures), other than that related to substance use, that can reasonably be presumed to be responsible for the clinical manifestations described under criterion A.

F1*x*.7 Residual and late-onset psychotic disorder

A. Conditions and disorders meeting the criteria for the individual syndromes listed below should be clearly related to substance use. Where onset of the condition or disorder occurs subsequent to use of psychoactive substances, strong evidence should be provided to demonstrate a link.

Comments

In view of the considerable variation in this category, the characteristics of such residual states or conditions should be clearly documented in terms of their type, severity, and duration. For research purposes full descriptive details should be specified.

A fifth character may be used, if required, as follows:

F1*x*.70 Flashbacks

F1*x*.71 Personality or behaviour disorder

B. The general criteria for F07.–, personality and behavioural disorder due to brain disease, damage and dysfunction, must be met.

F1*x*.72 Residual affective disorder

B. The criteria for F06.3, organic mood [affective] disorder, must be met.

F1*x*.73 Dementia

B. The general criteria for dementia (F00–F03) must be met.

F1*x*.74 Other persisting cognitive impairment

B. The criteria for F06.7, mild cognitive disorder, must be met, except for the exclusion of psychoactive substance use in criterion D.

F1*x*.75 Late-onset psychotic disorder

B. The general criteria for F1*x*.5, psychotic disorder, must be met, except with regard to the onset of the disorder, which is more than 2 weeks but not more than 6 weeks after substance use.

F1*x*.8 Other mental and behavioural disorders

F1*x*.9 Unspecified mental and behavioural disorder

F20 – F29
Schizophrenia, schizotypal and delusional disorders

F20 Schizophrenia

This overall category includes the common varieties of schizophrenia, together with some less common varieties and closely related disorders.

F20.0–F20.3 General criteria for paranoid, hebephrenic, catatonic, and undifferentiated schizophrenia

G1. Either *at least one* of the syndromes, symptoms, and signs listed under (1) below, *or* at least two of the symptoms and signs listed under (2) should be present for most of the time during an episode of psychotic illness lasting for at least 1 month (or at some time during most of the days).

(1) At least one of the following must be present:

(a) thought echo, thought insertion or withdrawal, or thought broadcasting;

(b) delusions of control, influence, or passivity, clearly referred to body or limb movements or specific thoughts, actions, or sensations; delusional perception;

(c) hallucinatory voices giving a running commentary on the patient's behaviour, or discussing the patient among themselves, or other types of hallucinatory voices coming from some part of the body;

(d) persistent delusions of other kinds that are culturally inappropriate and completely impossible (e.g. being able to control the weather, or being in communication with aliens from another world).

(2) *Or* at least two of the following:

(a) persistent hallucinations in any modality, when occurring every day for at least 1 month, when accompanied by delusions (which may be fleeting or half-formed) without clear affective content, or when accompanied by persistent over-valued ideas;

(b) neologisms, breaks, or interpolations in the train of thought, resulting in incoherence or irrelevant speech;

(c) catatonic behaviour, such as excitement, posturing or waxy flexibility, negativism, mutism, and stupor;

(d) "negative" symptoms, such as marked apathy, paucity of speech, and blunting or incongruity of emotional responses (it must be clear that these are not due to depression or to neuroleptic medication).

G2. *Most commonly used exclusion clauses*

(1) If the patient also meets criteria for manic episode (F30.–) or depressive episode (F32.–), the criteria listed under G1(1) and G1(2) above must have been met *before* the disturbance of mood developed.

(2) The disorder is not attributable to organic brain disease (in the sense of F00–F09), or to alcohol- or drug-related intoxication (F1*x*.0), dependence (F1*x*.2), or withdrawal (F1*x*.3 and F1*x*.4).

Comments

In evaluating the presence of these abnormal subjective experiences and behaviour, special care should be taken to avoid false-positive assessments, especially where culturally or subculturally influenced modes of expression and behaviour or a subnormal level of intelligence are involved.

Pattern of course

In view of the considerable variation of the course of schizophrenic disorders it may be desirable (especially for research) to specify the *pattern of course* by using a fifth character. Course should not usually be coded unless there has been a period of observation of at least 1 year. (For remission, see note 5 in Notes for users.)

F20.*x*0 Continuous

No remission of psychotic symptoms throughout the period of observation.

F20.*x*1 Episodic with progressive deficit

Progressive development of "negative" symptoms in the intervals between psychotic episodes.

F20.*x*2 Episodic with stable deficit

Persistent but non-progressive "negative" symptoms in the intervals between psychotic episodes.

F20.*x*3 Episodic remittent

Complete or virtually complete remissions between psychotic episodes.

F20.*x*4 Incomplete remission

F20.*x*5 Complete remission

F20.*x*8 Other

F20.*x*9 Course uncertain, period of observation too short

F20.0 Paranoid schizophrenia

A. The general criteria for schizophrenia (F20.0–F20.3) must be met.

B. Delusions or hallucinations must be prominent (such as delusions of persecution, reference, exalted birth, special mission, bodily change, or jealousy; threatening or commanding voices, hallucinations of smell or taste, sexual or other bodily sensations).

C. Flattening or incongruity of affect, catatonic symptoms, or incoherent speech must not dominate the clinical picture, although they may be present to a mild degree.

F20.1 Hebephrenic schizophrenia

A. The general criteria for schizophrenia (F20.0–F20.3) must be met.

B. Either of the following must be present:

(1) definite and sustained flattening or shallowness of affect;

(2) definite and sustained incongruity or inappropriateness of affect.

C. Either of the following must be present:

(1) behaviour that is aimless and disjointed rather than goal-directed;

(2) definite thought disorder, manifesting as speech that is disjointed, rambling, or incoherent.

D. Hallucinations or delusions must not dominate the clinical picture, although they may be present to a mild degree.

F20.2 Catatonic schizophrenia

A. The general criteria for schizophrenia (F20.0–F20.3) must eventually be met, although this may not be possible initially if the patient is uncommunicative.

B. For a period of at least 2 weeks one or more of the following catatonic behaviours must be prominent:

(1) stupor (marked decrease in reactivity to the environment anc reduction of spontaneous movements and activity) o mutism;

(2) excitement (apparently purposeless motor activity, not influ enced by external stimuli);

(3) posturing (voluntary assumption and maintenance of ina propriate or bizarre postures);

(4) negativism (an apparently motiveless resistance to all instru tions or attempts to be moved, or movement in the oppos direction);

(5) rigidity (maintenance of a rigid posture against efforts to moved);

(6) waxy flexibility (maintenance of limbs and body in externa imposed positions);

(7) command automatism (automatic compliance with instru tions).

F20.3 Undifferentiated schizophrenia

A. The general criteria for schizophrenia (F20.0–F20.3) must be m

B. Either of the following must apply:

(1) insufficient symptoms to meet the criteria for any of t subtypes F20.0, F20.1, F20.2, F20.4, or F20.5;

(2) so many symptoms that the criteria for more than one of tl subtypes listed in (1) above are met.

F20.4 Post-schizophrenic depression

A. The general criteria for schizophrenia (F20.0–F20.3) must hav been met within the past 12 months, but are not met at the preser time.

B. One of the conditions in criterion G1(2) a, b, c. or d fo F20.0–F20.3 must still be present.

C. The depressive symptoms must be sufficiently prolonged, severe, and extensive to meet criteria for at least a mild depressive episode (F32.0).

F20.5 Residual schizophrenia

A. The general criteria for schizophrenia (F20.0–F20.3) must have been met at some time in the past, but are not met at the present time.

B. At least four of the following "negative" symptoms have been present throughout the previous 12 months:

(1) psychomotor slowing or underactivity;

(2) definite blunting of affect;

(3) passivity and lack of initiative;

(4) poverty of either the quantity or the content of speech;

(5) poor non-verbal communication by facial expression, eye contact, voice modulation, or posture;

(6) poor social performance or self-care.

F20.6 Simple schizophrenia

A. There is slow but progressive development, over a period of at least 1 year, of all three of the following:

(1) a significant and consistent change in the overall quality of some aspects of personal behaviour, manifest as loss of drive and interests, aimlessness, idleness, a self-absorbed attitude, and social withdrawal;

(2) gradual appearance and deepening of "negative" symptoms such as marked apathy, paucity of speech, under-activity, blunting of affect, passivity and lack of initiative, and poor non-verbal communication (by facial expression, eye contact, voice modulation, and posture);

(3) marked decline in social, scholastic, or occupational performance.

B. At no time are there any of the symptoms referred to in criterion G1 for F20.0–F20.3, nor are there hallucinations or well formed delusions of any kind, i.e. the individual must never have met the criteria for any other type of schizophrenia or for any other psychotic disorder.

C. There is no evidence of dementia or any other organic mental disorder listed in F00–F09.

F20.8 Other schizophrenia

F20.9 Schizophrenia, unspecified

F21 Schizotypal disorder

A. The subject must have manifested at least four of the following over a period of at least 2 years, either continuously or repeatedly:

(1) inappropriate or constricted affect, with the individual appearing cold and aloof;

(2) behaviour or appearance that is odd, eccentric, or peculiar;

(3) poor rapport with others and a tendency to social withdrawal;

(4) odd beliefs or magical thinking, influencing behaviour and inconsistent with subcultural norms;

(5) suspiciousness or paranoid ideas;

(6) ruminations without inner resistance, often with dysmorphophobic, sexual, or aggressive contents;

(7) unusual perceptual experiences including somatosensory (bodily) or other illusions, depersonalization, or derealization;

(8) vague, circumstantial, metaphorical, overelaborate, or often stereotyped thinking, manifested by odd speech or in other ways, without gross incoherence;

(9) occasional transient quasi-psychotic episodes with intense illusions, auditory or other hallucinations, and delusion-like ideas, usually occurring without external provocation.

B. The subject must never have met the criteria for any disorder in F20.– (schizophrenia).

F22 Persistent delusional disorders

F22.0 Delusional disorder

A. A delusion or a set of related delusions, other than those listed as typically schizophrenic in criterion G1(1)b or d for F20.0–F20.3 (i.e. other than completely impossible or culturally inappropriate), must be present. The commonest examples are persecutory, grandiose, hypochondriacal, jealous (zelotypic), or erotic delusions.

B. The delusion(s) in criterion A must be present for at least 3 months.

C. The general criteria for schizophrenia (F20.0–F20.3) are not fulfilled.

D. There must be no persistent hallucinations in any modality (but there may be transitory or occasional auditory hallucinations that are not in the third person or giving a running commentary).

E. Depressive symptoms (or even a depressive episode (F32.–)) may be present intermittently, provided that the delusions persist at times when there is no disturbance of mood.

F. *Most commonly used exclusion clause.* There must be no evidence of primary or secondary organic mental disorder as listed under F00–F09, or of a psychotic disorder due to psychoactive substance use (F1*x*.5).

Specification for possible subtypes

The following types may be specified if desired: persecutory; litiginous; self-referential; grandiose; hypochondriacal (somatic); jealous; erotomanic.

F22.8 Other persistent delusional disorders

This is a residual category for persistent delusional disorders that do not meet the criteria for delusional disorder (F22.0). Disorders in which delusions are accompanied by persistent hallucinatory voices or by schizophrenic symptoms that are insufficient to meet criteria for schizophrenia (F20.–) should be coded here. Delusional disorders that have lasted for less than 3 months should, however, be coded, at least temporarily, under F23.–.

F22.9 Persistent delusional disorder, unspecified

F23 Acute and transient psychotic disorders

G1. There is acute onset of delusions, hallucinations, incomprehensible or incoherent speech, or any combination of these. The time interval between the first appearance of any psychotic symptoms and the presentation of the fully developed disorder should not exceed 2 weeks.

G2. If transient states of perplexity, misidentification, or impairment of attention and concentration are present, they do not fulfil the criteria for organically caused clouding of consciousness as specified for F05.–, criterion A.

G3. The disorder does not meet the symptomatic criteria for manic episode (F30.–), depressive episode (F32.–), or recurrent depressive disorder (F33.–).

G4. There is insufficient evidence of recent psychoactive substance use to fulfil the criteria for intoxication (F1*x*.0), harmful use (F1*x*.1), dependence (F1*x*.2), or withdrawal states (F1*x*.3 and F1*x*.4). The continued moderate and largely unchanged use of alcohol or drugs in amounts or with the frequency to which the individual is accustomed does not necessarily rule out the use of F23; this must be decided by clinical judgement and the requirements of the research project in question.

G5. *Most commonly used exclusion clause*. There must be no organic mental disorder (F00–F09) or serious metabolic disturbances affecting the central nervous system (this does not include childbirth).

A fifth character should be used to specify whether the acute onset of the disorder is associated with acute stress (occurring 2 weeks or less before evidence of first psychotic symptoms):

F23.*x*0 Without associated acute stress

F23.*x*1 With associated acute stress

For research purposes it is recommended that change of the disorder from a non-psychotic to a clearly psychotic state is further specified as either abrupt (onset within 48 hours) or acute (onset in more than 48 hours but less than 2 weeks).

F23.0 Acute polymorphic psychotic disorder without symptoms of schizophrenia

A. The general criteria for acute and transient psychotic disorders (F23) must be met.

B. Symptoms change rapidly in both type and intensity from day to day or within the same day.

C. Any type of either hallucinations or delusions occurs, for at least several hours, at any time from the onset of the disorder.

D. Symptoms from at least two of the following categories occur at the same time:

(1) emotional turmoil, characterized by intense feelings of happiness or ecstasy, or overwhelming anxiety or marked irritability;

(2) perplexity, or misidentification of people or places;

(3) increased or decreased motility, to a marked degree.

E. If any of the symptoms listed for schizophrenia (F20.0–F20.3), criterion G(1) and (2), are present, they are present only for a minority of the time from the onset, i.e. criterion B of F23.1 is not fulfilled.

F. The total duration of the disorder does not exceed 3 months.

F23.1 Acute polymorphic psychotic disorder with symptoms of schizophrenia

A. Criteria A, B, C, and D of acute polymorphic psychotic disorder (F23.0) must be met.

B. Some of the symptoms for schizophrenia (F20.0–F20.3) must have been present for the majority of the time since the onset of the disorder, although the full criteria need not be met, i.e. at least one of the symptoms in criteria G1(1)a to G1(2)c.

C. The symptoms of schizophrenia in criterion B above do not persist for more than 1 month.

F23.2 Acute schizophrenia-like psychotic disorder

A. The general criteria for acute and transient psychotic disorders (F23) must be met.

B. The criteria for schizophrenia (F20.0–F20.3) are met, with the exception of the criterion for duration.

C. The disorder does not meet criteria B, C, and D for acute polymorphic psychotic disorder (F23.0).

D. The total duration of the disorder does not exceed 1 month.

F23.3 Other acute predominantly delusional psychotic disorders

A. The general criteria for acute and transient psychotic disorders (F23) must be met.

B. Relatively stable delusions and/or hallucinations are present but do not fulfil the symptomatic criteria for schizophrenia (F20.0–F20.3).

C. The disorder does not meet the criteria for acute polymorphic psychotic disorder (F23.0).

D. The total duration of the disorder does not exceed 3 months.

F23.8 Other acute and transient psychotic disorders

Any other acute psychotic disorders that are not classifiable under any other category in F23 (such as acute psychotic states in which definite delusions or hallucinations occur but persist for only small proportions of the time) should be coded here. States of undifferentiated excitement should also be coded here if more detailed information about the patient's mental state is not available, provided that there is no evidence of an organic cause.

F23.9 Acute and transient psychotic disorder, unspecified

F24 Induced delusional disorder

A. The individual(s) must develop a delusion or delusional system originally held by someone else with a disorder classified in F20–F23.

B. The people concerned must have an unusually close relationship with one another, and be relatively isolated from other people.

C. The individual(s) must not have held the belief in question before contact with the other person, and must not have suffered from any other disorder classified in F20–F23 in the past.

F25 Schizoaffective disorders

Note. This diagnosis depends upon an approximate "balance" between the number, severity, and duration of the schizophrenic and affective symptoms.

G1. The disorder meets the criteria for one of the affective disorders (F30.–, F31.–, F32.–) of moderate or severe degree, as specified for each category.

G2. Symptoms from at least one of the groups listed below must be clearly present for most of the time during a period of at least 2 weeks (these groups are almost the same as for schizophrenia (F20.0–F20.3)):

(1) thought echo, thought insertion or withdrawal, thought broadcasting (criterion G1(1)a for F20.0–F20.3);

(2) delusions of control, influence, or passivity, clearly referred to body or limb movements or specific thoughts, actions, or sensations (criterion G1(1)b for F20.0–F20.3);

(3) hallucinatory voices giving a running commentary on the patient's behaviour or discussing the patient among themselves, or other types of hallucinatory voices coming from some part of the body (criterion G1(1)c for F20.0–F20.3);

(4) persistent delusions of other kinds that are culturally inappropriate and completely impossible, but not merely grandiose or persecutory (criterion G1(1)d for F20.0–F20.3), e.g. has visited other worlds; can control the clouds by breathing in and out; can communicate with plants or animals without speaking;

(5) grossly irrelevant or incoherent speech, or frequent use of neologisms (a marked form of criterion G1(2)b for F20.0–F20.3);

(6) intermittent but frequent appearance of some forms of catatonic behaviour, such as posturing, waxy flexibility, and negativism (criterion G1(2)c for F20.0–F20.3).

G3. Criteria G1 and G2 above must be met within the same episode of the disorder, and concurrently for at least part of the episode. Symptoms from both G1 and G2 must be prominent in the clinical picture.

G4. *Most commonly used exclusion clause.* The disorder is not attributable to organic mental disorder (in the sense of F00–F09), or to psychoactive substance-related intoxication, dependence, or withdrawal (F10–F19).

F25.0 Schizoaffective disorder, manic type

A. The general criteria for schizoaffective disorder (F25) must be met.

B. Criteria for a manic disorder (F30.1 or F31.1) must be met.

F25.1 Schizoaffective disorder, depressive type

A. The general criteria for schizoaffective disorder (F25) must be met.

B. The criteria for a depressive disorder of at least moderate severity (F31.3, F31.4, F32.1 or F32.2) must be met.

F25.2 Schizoaffective disorder, mixed type

A. The general criteria for schizoaffective disorder (F25) must be met.

B. The criteria for mixed bipolar affective disorder (F31.6) must be met.

F25.8 Other schizoaffective disorders

F25.9 Schizoaffective disorder, unspecified

Comments

If desired, further subtypes of schizoaffective disorder may be specified, according to the longitudinal development of the disorder, as follows:

F25.*x*0 Concurrent affective and schizophrenic symptoms only
Symptoms as defined in criterion G2 for F25.

F25.*x*1 Concurrent affective and schizophrenic symptoms, plus persistence of schizophrenic symptoms beyond the duration of affective symptoms

F28 Other nonorganic psychotic disorders

Psychotic disorders that do not meet the criteria for schizophrenia (F20.0–F20.3) or for psychotic types of mood [affective] disorders (F30–F39), and psychotic disorders that do not meet the symptomatic criteria for persistent delusional disorder (F22.–) should be coded here (persistent hallucinatory disorder is an example). Combinations of symptoms not covered by the previous categories F20–F25, such as delusions other than those listed as typically schizophrenic under criterion G1(1)b or d for F20.0–F20.3 (i.e. other than completely impossible or culturally inappropriate) plus catatonia, should also be included here.

F29 Unspecified nonorganic psychosis

F30 – F39
Mood [affective] disorders

F30 Manic episode

F30.0 Hypomania

A. The mood is elevated or irritable to a degree that is definitely abnormal for the individual concerned and sustained for at least 4 consecutive days.

B. At least three of the following signs must be present, leading to some interference with personal functioning in daily living:

(1) increased activity or physical restlessness;

(2) increased talkativeness;

(3) distractibility or difficulty in concentration;

(4) decreased need for sleep;

(5) increased sexual energy;

(6) mild over-spending, or other types of reckless or irresponsible behaviour;

(7) increased sociability or over-familiarity.

C. The episode does not meet the criteria for mania (F30.1 and F30.2), bipolar affective disorder (F31.–), depressive episode (F32.–), cyclothymia (F34.0), or anorexia nervosa (F50.0).

D. *Most commonly used exclusion clause.* The episode is not attributable to psychoactive substance use (F10–F19) or to any organic mental disorder (in the sense of F00–F09).

F30.1 Mania without psychotic symptoms

A. Mood must be predominantly elevated, expansive, or irritable, and definitely abnormal for the individual concerned. The mood change must be prominent and sustained for at least 1 week (unless it is severe enough to require hospital admission).

B. At least three of the following signs must be present (four if the mood is merely irritable), leading to severe interference with personal functioning in daily living:

(1) increased activity or physical restlessness;
(2) increased talkativeness ("pressure of speech");
(3) flight of ideas or the subjective experience of thoughts racing;
(4) loss of normal social inhibitions, resulting in behaviour that is inappropriate to the circumstances;
(5) decreased need for sleep;
(6) inflated self-esteem or grandiosity;
(7) distractibility or constant changes in activity or plans;
(8) behaviour that is foolhardy or reckless and whose risks the individual does not recognize, e.g. spending sprees, foolish enterprises, reckless driving;
(9) marked sexual energy or sexual indiscretions.

C. There are no hallucinations or delusions, although perceptual disorders may occur (e.g. subjective hyperacusis, appreciation of colours as especially vivid).

D. *Most commonly used exclusion clause*. The episode is not attributable to psychoactive substance use (F10–F19) or to any organic mental disorder (in the sense of F00–F09).

F30.2 Mania with psychotic symptoms

A. The episode meets the criteria for mania without psychotic symptoms (F30.1) with the exception of criterion C.

B. The episode does not simultaneously meet the criteria for schizophrenia (F20.0–F20.3) or schizoaffective disorder, manic type (F25.0).

C. Delusions or hallucinations are present, other than those listed as typically schizophrenic in criterion G1(1)b, c and d for F20.0–F20.3 (i.e. delusions other than those that are completely impossible or culturally inappropriate, and hallucinations that are not in the third person or giving a running commentary). The commonest examples are those with grandiose, self-referential, erotic, or persecutory content.

D. *Most commonly used exclusion clause*. The episode is not attributable to psychoactive substance use (F10–F19) or to any organic mental disorder (in the sense of F00–F09).

A fifth character may be used to specify whether the hallucinations or delusions are congruent or incongruent with the mood:

F30.20 With mood-congruent psychotic symptoms
(such as grandiose delusions or voices telling the individual that he or she has superhuman powers)

F30.21 With mood-incongruent psychotic symptoms
(such as voices speaking to the individual about affectively neutral topics, or delusions of reference or persecution)

F30.8 Other manic episodes

F30.9 Manic episode, unspecified

F31 Bipolar affective disorder

Note. Episodes are demarcated by a switch to an episode of opposite or mixed polarity or by a remission.

F31.0 Bipolar affective disorder, current episode hypomanic

A. The current episode meets the criteria for hypomania (F30.0).

B. There has been at least one other affective episode in the past, meeting the criteria for hypomanic or manic episode (F30.–), depressive episode (F32.–), or mixed affective episode (F38.00).

F31.1 Bipolar affective disorder, current episode manic without psychotic symptoms

A. The current episode meets the criteria for mania without psychotic symptoms (F30.1).

B. There has been at least one other affective episiode in the past, meeting the criteria for hypomanic or manic episode (F30.–), depressive episode (F32.–), or mixed affective episode (F38.00).

F31.2 Bipolar affective disorder, current episode manic with psychotic symptoms

A. The current episode meets the criteria for mania with psychotic symptoms (F30.2).

B. There has been at least one other affective episode in the past, meeting the criteria for hypomanic or manic episode (F30.–), depressive episode (F32.–), or mixed affective episode (F38.00).

A fifth character may be used to specify whether the psychotic symptoms are congruent or incongruent with the mood:

F31.20 With mood-congruent psychotic symptoms

F31.21 With mood-incongruent psychotic symptoms

F31.3 Bipolar affective disorder, current episode moderate or mild depression

A. The current episode meets the criteria for a depressive episode of either mild (F32.0) or moderate (F32.1) severity.

B. There has been at least one other affective episode in the past, meeting the criteria for hypomanic or manic episode (F30.–) or mixed affective episode (F38.00).

A fifth character may be used to specify the presence of the "somatic syndrome", as defined in F32.–, in the current episode of depression:

F31.30 Without somatic syndrome

F31.31 With somatic syndrome

F31.4 Bipolar affective disorder, current episode severe depression without psychotic symptoms

A. The current episode meets the criteria for a severe depressive episode without psychotic symptoms (F32.2).

B. There has been at least one well authenticated hypomanic or manic episode (F30.–) or mixed affective episode (F38.00) in the past.

F31.5 Bipolar affective disorder, current episode severe depression with psychotic symptoms

A. The current episode meets the criteria for a severe depressive episode with psychotic symptoms (F32.3).

B. There has been at least one well authenticated hypomanic or manic episode (F30.–) or mixed affective episode (F38.00) in the past.

A fifth character may be used to specify whether the psychotic symptoms are congruent or incongruent with the mood:

F31.50 With mood-congruent psychotic symptoms

F31.51 With mood-incongruent psychotic symptoms

F31.6 Bipolar affective disorder, current episode mixed

A. The current episode is characterized by either a mixture or a rapid alternation (i.e. within a few hours) of hypomanic, manic, and depressive symptoms.

B. Both manic and depressive symptoms must be prominent most of the time during a period of at least 2 weeks.

C. There has been at least one well authenticated hypomanic or manic episode (F30.–), depressive episode (F32.–), or mixed affective episode (F38.00) in the past.

F31.7 Bipolar affective disorder, currently in remission

A. The current state does not meet the criteria for depressive or manic episode of any severity or for any other mood disorder in F30–F39 (possibly because of treatment to reduce the risk of future episodes).

B. There has been at least one well authenticated hypomanic or manic episode (F30.–) in the past and in addition at least one other affective episode (hypomanic or manic (F30.–), depressive (F32.–), or mixed (F38.00)).

F31.8 Other bipolar affective disorders

F31.9 Bipolar affective disorder, unspecified

F32 Depressive episode

G1. The depressive episode should last for at least 2 weeks.

G2. There have been no hypomanic or manic symptoms sufficient to meet the criteria for hypomanic or manic episode (F30.–) at any time in the individual's life.

G3. *Most commonly used exclusion clause.* The episode is not attributable to psychoactive substance use (F10–F19) or to any organic mental disorder (in the sense of F00–F09).

Somatic syndrome

Some depressive symptoms are widely regarded as having special clinical significance and are here called "somatic". (Terms such as biological, vital, melancholic, or endogenomorphic are used for this syndrome in other classifications.)

A fifth character (as indicated in F31.3; F32.0 and F32.1; F33.0 and F33.1) may be used to specify the presence or absence of the somatic syndrome. To qualify for the somatic syndrome, *four* of the following symptoms should be present:

(1) marked loss of interest or pleasure in activities that are normally pleasurable;

(2) lack of emotional reactions to events or activities that normally produce an emotional response;

(3) waking in the morning 2 hours or more before the usual time;

(4) depression worse in the morning;

(5) objective evidence of marked psychomotor retardation or agitation (remarked on or reported by other people);

(6) marked loss of appetite;

(7) weight loss (5% or more of body weight in the past month);

(8) marked loss of libido.

In *The ICD-10 Classification of Mental and Behavioural Disorders: Clinical descriptions and diagnostic guidelines*, the presence or absence of the somatic syndrome is not specified for severe depressive episode, since it is presumed to be present in most cases. For research purposes, however, it may be advisable to allow for the coding of the absence of the somatic syndrome in severe depressive episode.

F32.0 Mild depressive episode

A. The general criteria for depressive episode (F32) must be met.

B. At least two of the following three symptoms must be present:

(1) depressed mood to a degree that is definitely abnormal for the individual, present for most of the day and almost every day,

largely uninfluenced by circumstances, and sustained for at least 2 weeks;

(2) loss of interest or pleasure in activities that are normally pleasurable;

(3) decreased energy or increased fatiguability.

C. An additional symptom or symptoms from the following list should be present, to give a total of at least *four*:

(1) loss of confidence or self-esteem;

(2) unreasonable feelings of self-reproach or excessive and inappropriate guilt;

(3) recurrent thoughts of death or suicide, or any suicidal behaviour;

(4) complaints or evidence of diminished ability to think or concentrate, such as indecisiveness or vacillation;

(5) change in psychomotor activity, with agitation or retardation (either subjective or objective);

(6) sleep disturbance of any type;

(7) change in appetite (decrease or increase) with corresponding weight change.

A fifth character may be used to specify the presence or absence of the "somatic syndrome" (defined on page 82):

F32.00 Without somatic syndrome

F32.01 With somatic syndrome

F32.1 Moderate depressive episode

A. The general criteria for depressive episode (F32) must be met.

B. At least two of the three symptoms listed for F32.0, criterion B, must be present.

C. Additional symptoms from F32.0, criterion C, must be present, to give a total of at least *six*.

A fifth character may be used to specify the presence or absence of the "somatic syndrome" (as defined on page 82):

F32.10 Without somatic syndrome

F32.11 With somatic syndrome

F32.2 Severe depressive episode without psychotic symptoms

Note: If important symptoms such as agitation or retardation are marked, the patient may be unwilling or unable to describe many symptoms in detail. An overall grading of severe episode may still be justified in such a case.

A. The general criteria for depressive episode (F32) must be met.

B. All three of the symptoms in criterion B, F32.0, must be present.

C. Additional symptoms from F32.0, criterion C, must be present, to give a total of at least *eight*.

D. There must be no hallucinations, delusions, or depressive stupor.

F32.3 Severe depressive episode with psychotic symptoms

A. The general criteria for depressive episode (F32) must be met.

B. The criteria for severe depressive episode without psychotic symptoms (F32.2) must be met with the exception of criterion D.

C. The criteria for schizophrenia (F20.0–F20.3) or schizoaffective disorder, depressive type (F25.1) are not met.

D. Either of the following must be present:
   (1) delusions or hallucinations, other than those listed as typically schizophrenic in criterion G1(1)b, c, and d for F20.0–F20.3 (i.e. delusions other than those that are completely impossible or culturally inappropriate and hallucinations that are not in the third person or giving a running commentary); the commonest examples are those with depressive, guilty, hypochondriacal, nihilistic, self-referential, or persecutory content;
   (2) depressive stupor.

A fifth character may be used to specify whether the psychotic symptoms are congruent or incongruent with mood:

F32.30 With mood-congruent psychotic symptoms

(i.e. delusions of guilt, worthlessness, bodily disease, or impending disaster, derisive or condemnatory auditory hallucinations)

F32.31 With mood-incongruent psychotic symptoms

(i.e. persecutory or self-referential delusions and hallucinations without an affective content)

F32.8 Other depressive episodes

Episodes should be included here which do not fit the descriptions given for depressive episodes in F32.0–F32.3, but for which the overall diagnostic impression indicates that they are depressive in nature. Examples include fluctuating mixtures of depressive symptoms (particularly those of the somatic syndrome) with non-diagnostic symptoms such as tension, worry, and distress, and mixtures of somatic depressive symptoms with persistent pain or fatigue not due to organic causes (as sometimes seen in general hospital services).

F32.9 Depressive episode, unspecified

F33 Recurrent depressive disorder

G1. There has been at least one previous episode, mild (F32.0), moderate (F32.1), or severe (F32.2 or F32.3), lasting a minimum of 2 weeks and separated from the current episode by at least 2 months free from any significant mood symptoms.

G2. At no time in the past has there been an episode meeting the criteria for hypomanic or manic episode (F30.–).

G3. *Most commonly used exclusion clause*. The episode is not attributable to psychoactive substance use (F10–F19) or to any organic mental disorder (in the sense of F00–F09).

It is recommended that the predominant type of previous episodes is specified (mild, moderate, severe, uncertain).

F33.0 Recurrent depressive disorder, current episode mild

A. The general criteria for recurrent depressive disorder (F33) are met.

B. The current episode meets the criteria for mild depressive episode (F32.0).

A fifth character may be used to specify the presence or absence of the "somatic syndrome", as defined on page 82, in the current episode:

F33.00 Without somatic syndrome

F33.01 With somatic syndrome

F33.1 Recurrent depressive disorder, current episode moderate

A. The general criteria for recurrent depressive disorder (F33) are met.

B. The current episode meets the criteria for moderate depressive episode (F32.1).

A fifth character may be used to specify the presence or absence of the "somatic syndrome," as defined on page 82, in the current episode:

F33.10 Without somatic syndrome

F33.11 With somatic syndrome

F33.2 Recurrent depressive disorder, current episode severe without psychotic symptoms

A. The general criteria for recurrent depressive disorder (F33) are met.

B. The current episode meets the criteria for severe depressive episode without psychotic symptoms (F32.2).

F33.3 Recurrent depressive disorder, current episode severe with psychotic symptoms

A. The general criteria for recurrent depressive disorder (F33) are met.

B. The current episode meets the criteria for severe depressive episode with psychotic symptoms (F32.3).

A fifth character may be used to specify whether the psychotic symptoms are congruent or incongruent with the mood:

F33.30 With mood-congruent psychotic symptoms

F33.31 With mood-incongruent psychotic symptoms

F33.4 Recurrent depressive disorder, currently in remission

A. The general criteria for recurrent depressive disorder (F33) have been met in the past.

B. The current state does not meet the criteria for a depressive episode (F32.–) of any severity or for any other disorder in F30–F39.

Comment

This category can still be used if the patient receives treatment to reduce the risk of further episodes.

F33.8 Other recurrent depressive disorders

F33.9 Recurrent depressive disorder, unspecified

F34 Persistent mood [affective] disorders

F34.0 Cyclothymia

A. There must have been a period of at least 2 years of instability of mood involving several periods of both depression and hypomania, with or without intervening periods of normal mood.

B. None of the manifestations of depression or hypomania during such a 2-year period should be sufficiently severe or long-lasting to meet criteria for manic episode or depressive episode (moderate or severe); however, manic or depressive episode(s) may have occurred before, or may develop after, such a period of persistent mood instability.

C. During at least some of the periods of depression at least three of the following should be present:

(1) reduced energy or activity;

(2) insomnia;

(3) loss of self-confidence or feelings of inadequacy;

(4) difficulty in concentrating;

(5) social withdrawal;

(6) loss of interest in or enjoyment of sex and other pleasurable activities;

(7) reduced talkativeness;

(8) pessimism about the future or brooding over the past.

D. During at least some of the periods of mood elevation at least three of the following should be present:

(1) increased energy or activity;

(2) decreased need for sleep;

(3) inflated self-esteem;

(4) sharpened or unusually creative thinking;

(5) increased gregariousness;

(6) increased talkativeness or wittiness;

(7) increased interest and involvement in sexual and other pleasurable activities;

(8) over-optimism or exaggeration of past achievements.

Note. If desired, time of onset may be specified as early (in late teenage or the twenties) or late (usually between age 30 and 50 years, following an affective episode).

F34.1 Dysthymia

A. There must be a period of at least 2 years of constant or constantly recurring depressed mood. Intervening periods of normal mood rarely last for longer than a few weeks and there are no episodes of hypomania.

B. None, or very few, of the individual episodes of depression within such a 2-year period should be sufficiently severe or long-lasting to meet the criteria for recurrent mild depressive disorder (F33.0).

C. During at least some of the periods of depression at least three of the following should be present:

(1) reduced energy or activity;

(2) insomnia;

(3) loss of self-confidence or feelings of inadequacy;

(4) difficulty in concentrating;

(5) frequent tearfulness;

(6) loss of interest in or enjoyment of sex and other pleasurable activities;

(7) feeling of hopelessness or despair;

(8) a perceived inability to cope with the routine responsibilities of everyday life;

(9) pessimism about the future or brooding over the past;

(10) social withdrawal;

(11) reduced talkativeness.

Note. If desired, time of onset may be specified as early (in late teenage or the twenties) or late (usually between age 30 and 50 years, following an affective episode).

F34.8 Other persistent mood [affective] disorders

This is a residual category for persistent affective disorders that are not sufficiently severe or long-lasting to fulfil the criteria for cyclothymia (F34.0) or dysthymia (F34.1) but that are nevertheless clinically significant. Some types of depression previously called "neurotic" are included here, provided that they do not meet the criteria for either cyclothymia (F34.0) or dysthymia (F34.1) or for depressive episode of mild (F32.0) or moderate (F32.1) severity.

F34.9 Persistent mood [affective] disorder, unspecified

F38 Other mood [affective] disorders

There are so many possible disorders that could be listed under F38 that no attempt has been made to specify criteria, except for mixed affective episode (F38.00) and recurrent brief depressive disorder (F38.10). Investigators requiring criteria more exact than those available in *Clinical descriptions and diagnostic guidelines* should construct them according to the requirements of their studies.

F38.0 Other single mood [affective] disorders

F38.00 Mixed affective episode

A. The episode is characterized by either a mixture or a rapid alternation (i.e. within a few hours) of hypomanic, manic, and depressive symptoms.

B. Both manic and depressive symptoms must be prominent most of the time during a period of at least 2 weeks.

C. There is no history of previous hypomanic, depressive, or mixed episodes.

F38.1 Other recurrent mood [affective] disorders

F38.10 Recurrent brief depressive disorder

A. The disorder meets the symptomatic criteria for mild (F32.0), moderate (F32.1), or severe (F32.2) depressive episode.

B. The depressive episodes have occurred about once a month over the past year.

C. The individual episodes last less than 2 weeks (typically 2–3 days).

D. The episodes do not occur solely in relation to the menstrual cycle.

F38.8 Other specified mood [affective] disorders

This is a residual category for affective disorders that do not meet the criteria for any other categories F30–F38.1 above.

F39 Unspecified mood [affective] disorder

F40 – F48
Neurotic, stress-related and somatoform disorders

F40 Phobic anxiety disorders

F40.0 Agoraphobia

A. There is marked and consistently manifest fear in, or avoidance of, at least two of the following situations:

(1) crowds;

(2) public places;

(3) travelling alone;

(4) travelling away from home.

B. At least two symptoms of anxiety in the feared situation must have been present together, on at least one occasion since the onset of the disorder, and one of the symptoms must have been from items (1) to (4) listed below:

Autonomic arousal symptoms

(1) palpitations or pounding heart, or accelerated heart rate;

(2) sweating;

(3) trembling or shaking;

(4) dry mouth (not due to medication or dehydration);

Symptoms involving chest and abdomen

(5) difficulty in breathing;

(6) feeling of choking;

(7) chest pain or discomfort;

(8) nausea or abdominal distress (e.g. churning in stomach);

Symptoms involving mental state

(9) feeling dizzy, unsteady, faint, or light-headed;

(10) feelings that objects are unreal (derealization), or that the self is distant or "not really here" (depersonalization);

(11) fear of losing control, "going crazy", or passing out;

(12) fear of dying;

General symptoms

(13) hot flushes or cold chills;

(14) numbness or tingling sensations.

C. Significant emotional distress is caused by the avoidance or by the anxiety symptoms, and the individual recognizes that these are excessive or unreasonable.

D. Symptoms are restricted to, or predominate in, the feared situations or contemplation of the feared situations.

E. *Most commonly used exclusion clause.* Fear or avoidance of situations (criterion A) is not the result of delusions, hallucinations, or other disorders such as organic mental disorders (F00–F09), schizophrenia and related disorders (F20–F29), mood [affective] disorders (F30–F39), or obsessive–compulsive disorder (F42.–), and is not secondary to cultural beliefs.

The presence or absence of panic disorder (F41.0) in a majority of agoraphobic situations may be specified by using a fifth character:

F40.00 Without panic disorder

F40.01 With panic disorder

Options for rating severity

Severity in F40.00 may be rated by indicating the degree of avoidance, taking into account the specific cultural setting. Severity in F40.01 may be rated by counting the number of panic attacks.

F40.1 Social phobias

A. Either of the following must be present:

(1) marked fear of being the focus of attention, or fear of behaving in a way that will be embarrassing or humiliating;

(2) marked avoidance of being the focus of attention, or of situations in which there is fear of behaving in an embarrassing or humiliating way.

These fears are manifested in social situations, such as eating or speaking in public, encountering known individuals in public, or entering or enduring small group situations (e.g. parties, meetings, classrooms).

B. At least two symptoms of anxiety in the feared situation as defined in F40.0, criterion B, must have been manifest at some time since the onset of the disorder, together with at least one of the following symptoms:

(1) blushing or shaking;

(2) fear of vomiting;

(3) urgency or fear of micturition or defecation.

C. Significant emotional distress is caused by the symptoms or by the avoidance, and the individual recognizes that these are excessive or unreasonable.

D. Symptoms are restricted to, or predominate in, the feared situations or contemplation of the feared situations.

E. *Most commonly used exclusion clause.* The symptoms listed in criteria A and B are not the result of delusions, hallucinations, or other disorders such as organic mental disorders (F00–F09), schizophrenia and related disorders (F20–F29), mood [affective] disorders (F30–F39), or obsessive–compulsive disorder (F42.–), and are not secondary to cultural beliefs.

F40.2 Specific (isolated) phobias

A. Either of the following must be present:

(1) marked fear of a specific object or situation not included in agoraphobia (F40.0) or social phobia (F40.1);

(2) marked avoidance of a specific object or situation not included in agoraphobia (F40.0) or social phobia (F40.1).

Among the most common objects and situations are animals, birds, insects, heights, thunder, flying, small enclosed spaces, the sight of blood or injury, injections, dentists, and hospitals.

B. Symptoms of anxiety in the feared situation as defined in F40.0, criterion B, must have been manifest at some time since the onset of the disorder.

C. Significant emotional distress is caused by the symptoms or by the avoidance, and the individual recognizes that these are excessive or unreasonable.

D. Symptoms are restricted to the feared situation or contemplation of the feared situation.

If desired, the specific phobias may be subdivided as follows:

— animal type (e.g. insects, dogs)
— nature-forces type (e.g. storms, water)
— blood, injection, and injury type
— situational type (e.g. elevators, tunnels)
— other type

F40.8 Other phobic anxiety disorders

F40.9 Phobic anxiety disorder, unspecified

F41 Other anxiety disorders

F41.0 Panic disorder [episodic paroxysmal anxiety]

A. The individual experiences recurrent panic attacks that are not consistently associated with a specific situation or object and that often occur spontaneously (i.e. the episodes are unpredictable). The panic attacks are not associated with marked exertion or with exposure to dangerous or life-threatening situations.

B. A panic attack is characterized by all of the following:

(1) it is a discrete episode of intense fear or discomfort;

(2) it starts abruptly;

(3) it reaches a maximum within a few minutes and lasts at least some minutes;

(4) at least four of the symptoms listed below must be present, one of which must be from items (a) to (d):

Autonomic arousal symptoms

(a) palpitations or pounding heart, or accelerated heart rate;
(b) sweating;
(c) trembling or shaking;
(d) dry mouth (not due to medication or dehydration);

Symptoms involving chest and abdomen

(e) difficulty in breathing;
(f) feeling of choking;
(g) chest pain or discomfort;
(h) nausea or abdominal distress (e.g. churning in stomach);

Symptoms involving mental state

(i) feeling dizzy, unsteady, faint, or light-headed;
(j) feelings that objects are unreal (derealization), or that the self is distant or "not really here" (depersonalization);
(k) fear of losing control, "going crazy", or passing out;
(l) fear of dying;

General symptoms

(m) hot flushes or cold chills;
(n) numbness or tingling sensations.

C. *Most commonly used exclusion clause.* Panic attacks are not due to a physical disorder, organic mental disorder (F00–F09), or other mental disorders such as schizophrenia and related disorders (F20–29), mood [affective] disorders (F30–39), or somatoform disorders (F45.–).

The range of individual variation in both content and severity is so great that two grades, moderate and severe, may be specified, if desired, with a fifth character:

F41.00 Panic disorder, moderate

At least four panic attacks in a 4-week period.

F41.01 Panic disorder, severe

At least four panic attacks per week over a 4-week period.

F41.1 Generalized anxiety disorder

Note. In children and adolescents the range of complaints by which the general anxiety is manifest is often more limited than in adults, and the specific symptoms of autonomic arousal are often less prominent. For these individuals, an alternative set of criteria is provided for use in F93.80 (generalized anxiety disorder of childhood), if preferred.

A. There must have been a period of at least 6 months with prominent tension, worry, and feelings of apprehension about everyday events and problems.

B. At least four of the symptoms listed below must be present, at least one of which must be from items (1) to (4):

Autonomic arousal symptoms

(1) palpitations or pounding heart, or accelerated heart rate;

(2) sweating;

(3) trembling or shaking;

(4) dry mouth (not due to medication or dehydration);

Symptoms involving chest and abdomen

(5) difficulty in breathing;

(6) feeling of choking;

(7) chest pain or discomfort;

(8) nausea or abdominal distress (e.g. churning in stomach);

Symptoms involving mental state

(9) feeling dizzy, unsteady, faint, or light-headed;

(10) feelings that objects are unreal (derealization), or that the self is distant or "not really here" (depersonalization);

(11) fear of losing control, "going crazy", or passing out;

(12) fear of dying;

General symptoms

(13) hot flushes or cold chills;

(14) numbness or tingling sensations;

Symptoms of tension

(15) muscle tension or aches and pains;

(16) restlessness and inability to relax;

(17) feeling keyed up, on edge, or mentally tense;

(18) a sensation of a lump in the throat, or difficulty in swallowing;

Other non-specific symptoms

(19) exaggerated response to minor surprises or being startled;

(20) difficulty in concentrating, or mind "going blank", because of worrying or anxiety;

(21) persistent irritability;

(22) difficulty in getting to sleep because of worrying.

C. The disorder does not meet the criteria for panic disorder (F41.0), phobic anxiety disorders (F40.–), obsessive–compulsive disorder (F42.–), or hypochondriacal disorder (F45.2).

D. *Most commonly used exclusion clause.* The anxiety disorder is not due to a physical disorder, such as hyperthyroidism, an organic mental disorder (F00–F09), or a psychoactive substance-related disorder (F10–F19), such as excess consumption of amfetamine-like substances or withdrawal from benzodiazepines.

F41.2 Mixed anxiety and depressive disorder

There are so many possible combinations of comparatively mild symptoms for these disorders that specific criteria are not given, other than those already in *Clinical descriptions and diagnostic guidelines.* It is suggested that researchers wishing to study patients with these disorders should arrive at their own criteria within the guidelines, depending upon the setting and purpose of their studies.

F41.3 Other mixed anxiety disorders

F41.8 Other specified anxiety disorders

F41.9 Anxiety disorder, unspecified

F42 Obsessive–compulsive disorder

A. Either obsessions or compulsions (or both) are present on most days for a period of at least 2 weeks.

B. Obsessions (thoughts, ideas, or images) and compulsions (acts) share the following features, all of which must be present:

(1) They are acknowledged as originating in the mind of the patient, and are not imposed by outside persons or influences.

(2) They are repetitive and unpleasant, and at least one obsession or compulsion that is acknowledged as excessive or unreasonable must be present.

(3) The patient tries to resist them (but resistance to very long-standing obsessions or compulsions may be minimal). At least one obsession or compulsion that is unsuccessfully resisted must be present.

(4) Experiencing the obsessive thought or carrying out the compulsive act is not in itself pleasurable. (This should be distinguished from the temporary relief of tension or anxiety.)

C. The obsessions or compulsions cause distress or interfere with the patient's social or individual functioning, usually by wasting time.

D. *Most commonly used exclusion clause*. The obsessions or compulsions are not the result of other mental disorders, such as schizophrenia and related disorders (F20–F29) or mood [affective] disorders (F30–F39).

The diagnosis may be further specified by the following four-character codes:

F42.0 Predominantly obsessional thoughts and ruminations

F42.1 Predominantly compulsive acts [obsessional rituals]

F42.2 Mixed obsessional thoughts and acts

F42.8 Other obsessive–compulsive disorders

F42.9 Obsessive–compulsive disorder, unspecified

F43 Reaction to severe stress, and adjustment disorders

F43.0 Acute stress reaction

A. The patient must have been exposed to an exceptional mental or physical stressor.

B. Exposure to the stressor is followed by an immediate onset of symptoms (within 1 hour).

C. Two groups of symptoms are given; the acute stress reaction is graded as:

F43.00 Mild

Only criterion (1) below is fulfilled.

F43.01 Moderate

Criterion (1) is met and there are any two symptoms from criterion (2).

F43.02 Severe

Either criterion (1) is met and there are any four symptoms from criterion (2); *or* there is dissociative stupor (see F44.2).

(1) Criteria B, C, and D for generalized anxiety disorder (F41.1) are met.

(2) (a) Withdrawal from expected social interaction.
(b) Narrowing of attention.
(c) Apparent disorientation.
(d) Anger or verbal aggression.
(e) Despair or hopelessness.
(f) Inappropriate or purposeless overactivity.
(g) Uncontrollable and excessive grief (judged by local cultural standards).

D. If the stressor is transient or can be relieved, the symptoms must begin to diminish after not more than 8 hours. If exposure to the stressor continues, the symptoms must begin to diminish after not more than 48 hours.

E. *Most commonly used exclusion clause*. The reaction must occur in the absence of any other concurrent mental or behavioural disorder in ICD-10 (except F41.1 (generalized anxiety disorder) and F60.– (personality disorders)), and not within 3 months of the end of an episode of any other mental or behavioural disorder.

F43.1 Post-traumatic stress disorder

A. The patient must have been exposed to a stressful event or situation (either short- or long-lasting) of exceptionally threatening or catastrophic nature, which would be likely to cause pervasive distress in almost anyone.

B. There must be persistent remembering or "reliving" of the stressor in intrusive "flashbacks", vivid memories, or recurring dreams, or in experiencing distress when exposed to circumstances resembling or associated with the stressor.

C. The patient must exhibit an actual or preferred avoidance of circumstances resembling or associated with the stressor, which was not present before exposure to the stressor.

D. Either of the following must be present:

(1) inability to recall, either partially or completely, some important aspects of the period of exposure to the stressor;

(2) persistent symptoms of increased psychological sensitivity and arousal (not present before exposure to the stressor), shown by any two of the following:

(a) difficulty in falling or staying asleep;

(b) irritability or outbursts of anger;

(c) difficulty in concentrating;

(d) hypervigilance;

(e) exaggerated startle response.

E. Criteria B, C, and D must all be met within 6 months of the stressful event or of the end of a period of stress. (For some purposes, onset delayed more than 6 months may be included, but this should be clearly specified.)

F43.2 Adjustment disorders

A. Onset of symptoms must occur within 1 month of exposure to an identifiable psychosocial stressor, not of an unusual or catastrophic type.

B. The individual manifests symptoms or behaviour disturbance of the types found in any of the affective disorders (F30–F39) (except for delusions and hallucinations), any disorders in F40–F48 (neurotic, stress-related, and somatoform disorders) and conduct disorders (F91.–), but the criteria for an individual disorder are not fulfilled. Symptoms may be variable in both form and severity.

The predominant feature of the symptoms may be further specified by the use of a fifth character:

F43.20 **Brief depressive reaction**

A transient mild depressive state of a duration not exceeding 1 month.

F43.21 **Prolonged depressive reaction**

A mild depressive state occurring in response to a prolonged exposure to a stressful situation but of a duration not exceeding 2 years.

F43.22 **Mixed anxiety and depressive reaction**

Both anxiety and depressive symptoms are prominent, but at levels no greater than those specified for mixed anxiety and depressive disorder (F41.2) or other mixed anxiety disorders (F41.3).

F43.23 **With predominant disturbance of other emotions**

The symptoms are usually of several types of emotion, such as anxiety, depression, worry, tensions, and anger. Symptoms of anxiety and depression may meet the criteria for mixed anxiety and depressive disorder (F41.2) or for other mixed anxiety disorders (F41.3), but they are not so predominant that other more specific depressive or anxiety disorders can be diagnosed. This category should also be used for reactions in children in whom regressive behaviour such as bed-wetting or thumb-sucking is also present.

F43.24 **With predominant disturbance of conduct**

The main disturbance is one involving conduct, e.g. an adolescent grief reaction resulting in aggressive or dissocial behaviour.

F43.25 **With mixed disturbance of emotions and conduct**

Both emotional symptoms and disturbances of conduct are prominent features.

F43.28 **With other specified predominant symptoms**

C. Except in prolonged depressive reaction (F43.21), the symptoms do not persist for more than 6 months after the cessation of the stress or its consequences. However, this should not prevent a provisional diagnosis being made if this criterion is not yet fulfilled.

F43.8 Other reactions to severe stress

F43.9 Reaction to severe stress, unspecified

F44 Dissociative [conversion] disorders

G1. There must be no evidence of a physical disorder that can explain the characteristic symptoms of this disorder (although physical disorders may be present that give rise to other symptoms).

G2. There are convincing associations in time between the onset of symptoms of the disorder and stressful events, problems, or needs.

F44.0 Dissociative amnesia

A. The general criteria for dissociative disorder (F44) must be met.

B. There must be amnesia, either partial or complete, for recent events or problems that were or still are traumatic or stressful.

C. The amnesia is too extensive and persistent to be explained by ordinary forgetfulness (although its depth and extent may vary from one assessment to the next) or by intentional simulation.

F44.1 Dissociative fugue

A. The general criteria for dissociative disorder (F44) must be met.

B. The individual undertakes an unexpected yet organized journey away from home or from the ordinary places of work and social activities, during which self-care is largely maintained.

C. There is amnesia, either partial or complete, for the journey, which also meets criterion C for dissociative amnesia (F44.0).

F44.2 Dissociative stupor

A. The general criteria for dissociative disorder (F44) must be met.

B. There is profound diminution or absence of voluntary movements and speech and of normal responsiveness to light, noise, and touch.

C. Normal muscle tone, static posture, and breathing (and often limited coordinated eye movements) are maintained.

F44.3 Trance and possession disorders

A. The general criteria for dissociative disorder (F44) must be met.

B. Either of the following must be present:

(1) *Trance*. There is temporary alteration of the state of consciousness, shown by any two of:

(a) loss of the usual sense of personal identity;

(b) narrowing of awareness of immediate surroundings, or unusually narrow and selective focusing on environmental stimuli;

(c) limitation of movements, postures, and speech to repetition of a small repertoire.

(2) *Possession disorder*. The individual is convinced that he or she has been taken over by a spirit, power, deity, or other person.

C. Both (1) and (2) of criterion B must be unwanted and troublesome, occurring outside, or being a prolongation of, similar states in religious or other culturally accepted situations.

D. *Most commonly used exclusion clause*. The disorder does not occur at the same time as schizophrenia or related disorders (F20–F29), or mood [affective] disorders (F30–F39) with hallucinations or delusions.

F44.4 Dissociative motor disorders

A. The general criteria for dissociative disorder (F44) must be met.

B. Either of the following must be present:

(1) complete or partial loss of the ability to perform movements that are normally under voluntary control (including speech);

(2) various or variable degrees of incoordination or ataxia, or inability to stand unaided.

F44.5 Dissociative convulsions

A. The general criteria for dissociative disorder (F44) must be met.

B. The individual exhibits sudden and unexpected spasmodic movements, closely resembling any of the varieties of epileptic seizure, but not followed by loss of consciousness.

C. The symptoms in criterion B are not accompanied by tongue-biting, serious bruising or laceration due to falling, or urinary incontinence.

F44.6 Dissociative anaesthesia and sensory loss

A. The general criteria for dissociative disorder (F44) must be met.

B. Either of the following must be present:

(1) partial or complete loss of any or all of the normal cutaneous sensations over part or all of the body (specify: touch, pin-prick, vibration, heat, cold);

(2) partial or complete loss of vision, hearing, or smell (specify).

F44.7 Mixed dissociative [conversion] disorders

F44.8 Other dissociative [conversion] disorders

This residual code may be used to indicate other dissociative and conversion states that meet criteria G1 and G2 for F44, but do not meet the criteria for F44.0–F44.7 listed above.

F44.80 Ganser's syndrome

(approximate answers)

F44.81 Multiple personality disorder

A. Two or more distinct personalities exist within the individual, only one being evident at a time.

B. Each personality has its own memories, preferences, and behaviour patterns, and at some time (and recurrently) takes full control of the individual's behaviour.

C. There is inability to recall important personal information which is too extensive to be explained by ordinary forgetfulness.

D. The symptoms are not due to organic mental disorders (F00–F09) (e.g. in epileptic disorders) or to psychoactive substance-related disorders (F10–F19) (e.g. intoxication or withdrawal).

F44.82 Transient dissociative [conversion] disorders occurring in childhood and adolescence

F44.88 Other specified dissociative [conversion] disorders

Specific research criteria are not given for all disorders mentioned above, since these other dissociative states are rare and not well described. Research workers studying these conditions in detail should specify their own criteria according to the purposes of their studies.

F44.9 Dissociative [conversion] disorder, unspecified

F45 Somatoform disorders

F45.0 Somatization disorder

A. There must be a history of at least 2 years' complaints of multiple and variable physical symptoms that cannot be explained by any detectable physical disorders. (Any physical disorders that are known to be present do not explain the severity, extent, variety, and persistence of the physical complaints, or the associated social disability.) If some symptoms clearly due to autonomic arousal are present, they are not a major feature of the disorder in that they are not particularly persistent or distressing.

B. Preoccupation with the symptoms causes persistent distress and leads the patient to seek repeated (three or more) consultations or sets of investigations with either primary care or specialist doctors. In the absence of medical services within either the financial or physical reach of the patient, there must be persistent self-medication or multiple consultations with local healers.

C. There is persistent refusal to accept medical reassurance that there is no adequate physical cause for the physical symptoms. (Short-term acceptance of such reassurance, i.e. for a few weeks during or immediately after investigations, does not exclude this diagnosis.)

D. There must be a total of six or more symptoms from the following list, with symptoms occurring in at least two separate groups:

Gastrointestinal symptoms

(1) abdominal pain;

(2) nausea;

(3) feeling bloated or full of gas;

(4) bad taste in mouth, or excessively coated tongue;

(5) complaints of vomiting or regurgitation of food;

(6) complaints of frequent and loose bowel motions or discharge of fluids from anus;

Cardiovascular symptoms

(7) breathlessness without exertion;

(8) chest pains;

Genitourinary symptoms

(9) dysuria or complaints of frequency of micturition;

(10) unpleasant sensations in or around the genitals;

(11) complaints of unusual or copious vaginal discharge;

Skin and pain symptoms

(12) blotchiness or discoloration of the skin;

(13) pain in the limbs, extremities, or joints;

(14) unpleasant numbness or tingling sensations.

E. *Most commonly used exclusion clause.* Symptoms do not occur only during any of the schizophrenic or related disorders (F20–F29), any of the mood [affective] disorders (F30–F39), or panic disorder (F41.0).

F45.1 Undifferentiated somatoform disorder

A. Criteria A, C, and E for somatization disorder (F45.0) are met, except that the duration of the disorder is at least 6 months.

B. One or both of criteria B and D for somatization disorder (F45.0) are incompletely fulfilled.

F45.2 Hypochondriacal disorder

A. Either of the following must be present:

(1) a persistent belief, of at least 6 months' duration, of the presence of a maximum of two serious physical diseases (of which at least one must be specifically named by the patient);

(2) a persistent preoccupation with a presumed deformity or disfigurement (body dysmorphic disorder).

B. Preoccupation with the belief and the symptoms causes persistent distress or interference with personal functioning in daily living, and leads the patient to seek medical treatment or investigations (or equivalent help from local healers).

C. There is persistent refusal to accept medical reassurance that there is no physical cause for the symptoms or physical abnormality. (Short-term acceptance of such reassurance, i.e. for a few weeks during or immediately after investigations, does not exclude this diagnosis.)

D. *Most commonly used exclusion clause.* The symptoms do not occur only during any of the schizophrenic and related disorders (F20–F29, particularly F22) or any of the mood [affective] disorders (F30–F39).

F45.3 Somatoform autonomic dysfunction

A. There must be symptoms of autonomic arousal that are attributed by the patient to a physical disorder of one or more of the following systems or organs:

(1) heart and cardiovascular system;

(2) upper gastrointestinal tract (oesophagus and stomach);

(3) lower gastrointestinal tract;

(4) respiratory system;

(5) genitourinary system.

B. Two or more of the following autonomic symptoms must be present:

(1) palpitations;

(2) sweating (hot or cold);

(3) dry mouth;

(4) flushing or blushing;

(5) epigastric discomfort, "butterflies", or churning in the stomach.

C. One or more of the following symptoms must be present:

(1) chest pains or discomfort in and around the precordium;

(2) dyspnoea or hyperventilation;

(3) excessive tiredness on mild exertion;

(4) aerophagy, hiccough, or burning sensations in chest or epigastrium;

(5) reported frequent bowel movements;

(6) increased frequency of micturition or dysuria;

(7) feeling of being bloated, distended, or heavy.

D. There is no evidence of a disturbance of structure or function in the organs or systems about which the patient is concerned.

E. *Most commonly used exclusion clause.* These symptoms do not occur only in the presence of phobic disorders (F40.0–F40.3) or panic disorder (F41.0).

A fifth character is to be used to classify the individual disorders in this group, indicating the organ or system regarded by the patient as the origin of the symptoms: .

F45.30 Heart and cardiovascular system
Includes: cardiac neurosis, neurocirculatory asthenia, Da Costa's syndrome.

F45.31 Upper gastrointestinal tract
Includes: psychogenic aerophagy, hiccough, gastric neurosis.

F45.32 Lower gastrointestinal tract
Includes: psychogenic irritable bowel syndrome, psychogenic diarrhoea, gas syndrome.

F45.33 Respiratory system
Includes: hyperventilation.

F45.34 Genitourinary system
Includes: psychogenic increase of frequency of micturition and dysuria.

F45.38 Other organ or system

F45.4 Persistent somatoform pain disorder

A. There is persistent severe and distressing pain (for at least 6 months, and continuously on most days), in any part of the body, which cannot be explained adequately by evidence of a physiological process or a physical disorder, and which is consistently the main focus of the patient's attention.

B. *Most commonly used exclusion clause.* This disorder does not occur in the presence of schizophrenia or related disorders (F20–F29), or only during any of the mood [affective] disorders (F30–F39), somatization disorder (F45.0), undifferentiated somatoform disorder (F45.1), or hypochondriacal disorder (F45.2).

F45.8 Other somatoform disorders

In these disorders the presenting complaints are not mediated through the autonomic nervous system, and are limited to specific systems or parts of the body, such as the skin. This is in contrast to the multiple and often changing complaints of the origin of symptoms and distress found in somatization disorder (F45.0) and undifferentiated somatoform disorder (F45.1). Tissue damage is not involved.

Any other disorders of sensation not due to physical disorders, which are closely associated in time with stressful events or problems, or which result in significantly increased attention for the patient, either personal or medical, should also be classified here.

F45.9 Somatoform disorder, unspecified

F48 Other neurotic disorders

F48.0 Neurasthenia

A. Either of the following must be present:

(1) persistent and distressing complaints of feelings of exhaustion after minor mental effort (such as performing or attempting to perform everyday tasks that do not require unusual mental effort);

(2) persistent and distressing complaints of feelings of fatigue and bodily weakness after minor physical effort.

B. At least one of the following symptoms must be present:

(1) feelings of muscular aches and pains;

(2) dizziness;

(3) tension headaches;

(4) sleep disturbance;

(5) inability to relax;

(6) irritability.

C. The patient is unable to recover from the symptoms in criterion A (1) or (2) by means of rest, relaxation, or entertainment.

D. The duration of the disorder is at least 3 months.

E. *Most commonly used exclusion clause.* The disorder does not occur in the presence of organic emotionally labile disorder (F06.6), postencephalitic syndrome (F07.1), postconcussional syndrome (F07.2), mood [affective] disorders (F30–F39), panic disorder (F41.0), or generalized anxiety disorder (F41.1).

F48.1 Depersonalization–derealization syndrome

A. Either of the following must be present:

(1) *Depersonalization.* The patient complains of a feeling of being distant or "not really here". For example, individuals may complain that their emotions, feelings, or experience of the inner self are detached, strange, not their own, or unpleasantly lost, or that their emotions or movements seem as if they belong to someone else, or that they feel as if acting in a play.

(2) *Derealization.* The patient complains of a feeling of unreality. For example, there may be complaints that the surroundings or specific objects look strange, distorted, flat, colourless, lifeless, dreary, uninteresting, or like a stage upon which everyone is acting.

B. There is retention of insight, in that the patient realizes that the change is not imposed from outside by other persons or forces.

Comments

This diagnosis should not be used as a main or single diagnosis when the syndrome arises in the presence of other mental disorders, such as organic confusional or delusional states (F05.–, F06.–), intoxication by alcohol or drugs (F1*x*.0), schizophrenia and related disorders (F20–F29), mood [affective] disorders (F30–F39), anxiety disorders (F40.–, F41.–), or other conditions (such as marked fatigue, hypoglycaemia, or immediately preceding or following epileptic seizures). However, these syndromes often occur during the course of many other psychiatric disorders, and are appropriately recorded as a secondary or additional diagnosis to a different main diagnosis. Their occurrence as isolated syndromes is much less common.

F48.8 Other specified neurotic disorders

This category includes mixed disorders of behaviour, beliefs, and emotions, which are of uncertain etiology and nosological status and which occur with particular frequency in certain cultures (see also Annex 2); examples include dhat syndrome (undue concern about the debilitating effects of the passage of semen), koro (anxiety and fear that the penis will retract into the abdomen and cause death), and latah (imitative and automatic response behaviour). The strong association of these syndromes with locally accepted cultural beliefs and patterns of behaviour indicates that they are probably best regarded as not delusional.

F48.9 Neurotic disorder, unspecified

F50 – F59
Behavioural syndromes associated with physiological disturbances and physical factors

F50 Eating disorders

F50.0 Anorexia nervosa

A. There is weight loss or, in children, a lack of weight gain, leading to a body weight at least 15% below the normal or expected weight for age and height.

B. The weight loss is self-induced by avoidance of "fattening foods".

C. There is self-perception of being too fat, with an intrusive dread of fatness, which leads to a self-imposed low weight threshold.

D. A widespread endocrine disorder involving the hypothalamic–pituitary–gonadal axis is manifest in women as amenorrhoea and in men as a loss of sexual interest and potency. (An apparent exception is the persistence of vaginal bleeds in anorexic women who are on replacement hormonal therapy, most commonly taken as a contraceptive pill.)

E. The disorder does not meet criteria A and B for bulimia nervosa (F50.2).

Comments

The following features support the diagnosis, but are not essential elements: self-induced vomiting, self-induced purging, excessive exercise, and use of appetite suppressants and/or diuretics.

If onset is prepubertal, the sequence of pubertal events is delayed or even arrested (growth ceases; in girls the breasts do not develop and there is a primary amenorrhoea; in boys the genitals remain juvenile). With recovery, puberty is often completed normally, but the menarche is late.

F50.1 Atypical anorexia nervosa

Researchers studying atypical forms of anorexia nervosa are recommended to make their own decisions about the number and type of criteria to be fulfilled.

F50.2 Bulimia nervosa

A. There are recurrent episodes of overeating (at least twice a week over a period of 3 months) in which large amounts of food are consumed in short periods of time.

B. There is persistent preoccupation with eating, and a strong desire or a sense of compulsion to eat (craving).

C. The patient attempts to counteract the "fattening" effects of food by one or more of the following:

(1) self-induced vomiting;

(2) self-induced purging;

(3) alternating periods of starvation;

(4) use of drugs such as appetite suppressants, thyroid preparations, or diuretics; when bulimia occurs in diabetic patients they may choose to neglect their insulin treatment.

D. There is self-perception of being too fat, with an intrusive dread of fatness (usually leading to underweight).

F50.3 Atypical bulimia nervosa

Researchers studying atypical forms of bulimia nervosa, such as those involving normal or excessive body weight, are recommended to make their own decisions about the number and type of criteria to be fulfilled.

F50.4 Overeating associated with other psychological disturbances

Researchers wishing to use this category are recommended to design their own criteria.

F50.5 Vomiting associated with other psychological disturbances

Researchers wishing to use this category are recommended to design their own criteria.

F50.8 Other eating disorders

F50.9 Eating disorder, unspecified

F51 Nonorganic sleep disorders

Note: A more comprehensive classification of sleep disorders is available (*International classification of sleep disorders*[1]) but it should be noted that this is organized differently from ICD-10.

For some research purposes, where particularly homogeneous groups of sleep disorders are required, four or more events occurring within a 1-year period may be considered as a criterion for use of categories F51.3, F51.4, and F51.5.

F51.0 Nonorganic insomnia

A. The individual complains of difficulty falling asleep, difficulty maintaining sleep, or non-refreshing sleep.

B. The sleep disturbance occurs at least three times a week for at least 1 month.

C. The sleep disturbance results in marked personal distress or interference with personal functioning in daily living.

D. There is no known causative organic factor, such as a neurological or other medical condition, psychoactive substance use disorder, or a medication.

F51.1 Nonorganic hypersomnia

A. The individual complains of excessive daytime sleepiness or sleep attacks or of prolonged transition to the fully aroused state upon awakening (sleep drunkenness), which is not accounted for by an inadequate amount of sleep.

B. This sleep disturbance occurs nearly every day for at least 1 month or recurrently for shorter periods of time, and causes either marked distress or interference with personal functioning in daily living.

C. There are no auxiliary symptoms of narcolepsy (cataplexy, sleep paralysis, hypnagogic hallucinations) and no clinical evidence for sleep apnoea (nocturnal breath cessation, typical intermittent snorting sounds, etc.).

---

[1] Diagnostic Classification Steering Committee. *International classification of sleep disorders: Diagnostic and coding manual*. Rochester, MN, American Sleep Disorders Association, 1990.

D. There is no known causative organic factor, such as a neurological or other medical condition, psychoactive substance use disorder, or a medication.

F51.2 Nonorganic disorder of the sleep–wake schedule

A. The individual's sleep–wake pattern is out of synchrony with the desired sleep–wake schedule, as imposed by societal demands and shared by most people in the individual's environment.

B. As a result of disturbance of the sleep–wake schedule, the individual experiences insomnia during the major sleep period or hypersomnia during the waking period, nearly every day for at least 1 month or recurrently for shorter periods of time.

C. The unsatisfactory quantity, quality, and timing of sleep causes either marked personal distress or interference with personal functioning in daily living.

D. There is no known causative organic factor, such as a neurological or other medical condition, psychoactive substance use disorder, or a medication.

F51.3 Sleepwalking [somnambulism]

A. The predominant symptom is repeated (two or more) episodes of rising from bed, usually during the first third of nocturnal sleep, and walking about for between several minutes and half an hour.

B. During an episode, the individual has a blank, staring face, is relatively unresponsive to the efforts of others to influence the event or to communicate with him or her, and can be awakened only with considerable difficulty.

C. Upon awakening (either from an episode or the next morning) the individual has amnesia for the episode.

D. Within several minutes of awakening from the episode, there is no impairment of mental activity or behaviour, although there may initially be a short period of some confusion and disorientation.

E. There is no evidence of an organic mental disorder, such as dementia, or a physical disorder, such as epilepsy.

F51.4 Sleep terrors [night terrors]

A. Repeated (two or more) episodes in which the individual gets up from sleep with a panicky scream and intense anxiety, body motility, and autonomic hyperactivity (such as tachycardia, heart pounding, rapid breathing, and sweating).

B. The episodes occur mainly during the first third of sleep.

C. The duration of the episode is less than 10 minutes.

D. If others try to comfort the individual during the episode, there is a lack of response followed by disorientation and perseverative movements.

E. The individual has limited recall of the event.

F. There is no known causative organic factor, such as a neurological or other medical condition, psychoactive substance use disorder, or a medication.

F51.5 Nightmares

A. The individual wakes from nocturnal sleep or naps with detailed and vivid recall of intensely frightening dreams, usually involving threats to survival, security, or self-esteem. The awakening may occur during any part of the sleep period, but typically during the second half.

B. Upon awakening from the frightening dreams, the individual rapidly becomes oriented and alert.

C. The dream experience itself and the disturbance of sleep resulting from the awakenings associated with the episodes cause marked distress to the individual.

D. There is no known causative organic factor, such as a neurological or other medical condition, psychoactive substance use disorder, or a medication.

F51.8 Other nonorganic sleep disorders

F51.9 Nonorganic sleep disorder, unspecified

F52 Sexual dysfunction, not caused by organic disorder or disease

G1. The subject is unable to participate in a sexual relationship as he or she would wish.

G2. The dysfunction occurs frequently, but may be absent on some occasions.

G3. The dysfunction has been present for at least 6 months.

G4. The dysfunction is not entirely attributable to any of the other mental and behavioural disorders in ICD-10, physical disorders (such as endocrine disorder), or drug treatment.

Comments

Measurement of each form of dysfunction can be based on rating scales that assess severity as well as frequency of the problem. More than one type of dysfunction can coexist.

F52.0 Lack or loss of sexual desire

A. The general criteria for sexual dysfunction (F52) must be met.

B. There is a lack or loss of sexual desire, manifest by diminution of seeking out sexual cues, of thinking about sex with associated feelings of desire or appetite, or of sexual fantasies.

C. There is a lack of interest in initiating sexual activity either with a partner or as solitary masturbation, resulting in a frequency of activity clearly lower than expected, taking into account age and context, or in a frequency very clearly reduced from previous much higher levels.

F52.1 Sexual aversion and lack of sexual enjoyment

F52.10 Sexual aversion

A. The general criteria for sexual dysfunction (F52) must be met.

B. The prospect of sexual interaction with a partner produces sufficient aversion, fear, or anxiety that sexual activity is avoided, or, if it occurs, is associated with strong negative feelings and an inability to experience any pleasure.

C. The aversion is not the result of performance anxiety (reaction to previous failure of sexual response).

F52.11 Lack of sexual enjoyment

A. The general criteria for sexual dysfunction (F52) must be met.

B. Genital response (orgasm and/or ejaculation) occurs during sexual stimulation, but is not accompanied by pleasurable sensations or feelings of pleasant excitement.

C. There is no manifest and persistent fear or anxiety during sexual activity (see F52.10, sexual aversion).

F52.2 Failure of genital response

A. The general criteria for sexual dysfunction (F52) must be met.

In addition, for men:

B. Erection sufficient for intercourse fails to occur when intercourse is attempted. The dysfunction takes one of the following forms:

(1) full erection occurs during the early stages of lovemaking but disappears or declines when intercourse is attempted (before ejaculation if it occurs);

(2) erection does occur, but only at times when intercourse is not being considered;

(3) partial erection, insufficient for intercourse, occurs, but not full erection;

(4) no penile tumescence occurs at all.

In addition, for women:

B. There is failure of genital response, experienced as failure of vaginal lubrication, together with inadequate tumescence of the labia. The dysfunction takes one of the following forms:

(1) general: lubrication fails in all relevant circumstances;

(2) lubrication may occur initially but fails to persist for long enough to allow comfortable penile entry;

(3) situational: lubrication occurs only in some situations (e.g. with one partner but not another, or during masturbation, or when vaginal intercourse is not being contemplated).

F52.3 Orgasmic dysfunction

A. The general criteria for sexual dysfunction (F52) must be met.

B. There is orgasmic dysfunction (either absence or marked delay of orgasm) which takes one of the following forms:

(1) orgasm has never been experienced in any situation;

(2) orgasmic dysfunction has developed after a period of relatively normal response:

(a) general: orgasmic dysfunction occurs in all situations and with any partner;

(b) situational:
for *women*: orgasm does occur in certain situations (e.g. when masturbating or with certain partners);

for *men*, one of the following can be applied:

i) orgasm occurs only during sleep, never during the waking state;
ii) orgasm never occurs in the presence of the partner;
iii) orgasm occurs in the presence of the partner but not during intercourse.

F52.4 Premature ejaculation

A. The general criteria for sexual dysfunction (F52) must be met.

B. There is an inability to delay ejaculation sufficiently to enjoy lovemaking, manifest as either of the following:

(1) occurrence of ejaculation before or very soon after the beginning of intercourse (if a time limit is required: before or within 15 seconds of the beginning of intercourse);

(2) ejaculation occurs in the absence of sufficient erection to make intercourse possible.

C. The problem is not the result of prolonged abstinence from sexual activity.

F52.5 Nonorganic vaginismus

A. The general criteria for sexual dysfunction (F52) must be met.

B. There is spasm of the perivaginal muscles, sufficient to prevent penile entry or make it uncomfortable. The dysfunction takes one of the following forms:

(1) normal response has never been experienced;

(2) vaginismus has developed after a period of relatively normal response:

(a) when vaginal entry is not attempted, a normal sexual response may occur;

(b) any attempt at sexual contact leads to generalized fear and efforts to avoid vaginal entry (e.g. spasm of the adductor muscles of the thighs).

F52.6 Nonorganic dyspareunia

A. The general criteria for sexual dysfunction (F52) must be met.

In addition, for women:

B. Pain is experienced at the entry of the vagina, either throughout sexual intercourse or only when deep thrusting of the penis occurs.

C. The disorder is not attributable to vaginismus or failure of lubrication; dyspareunia of organic origin should be classified according to the underlying disorder.

In addition, for men:

B. Pain or discomfort is experienced during sexual response. (The timing of the pain and the exact localization should be carefully recorded.)

C. The discomfort is not the result of local physical factors. If physical factors are found, the dysfunction should be classified elsewhere.

F52.7 Excessive sexual drive

No research criteria are attempted for this category. Researchers studying this category are recommended to design their own criteria.

F52.8 Other sexual dysfunction, not caused by organic disorder or disease

F52.9 Unspecified sexual dysfunction, not caused by organic disorder or disease

F53 Mental and behavioural disorders associated with the puerperium, not elsewhere classified

This category should be used in research work only in exceptional circumstances. Mental disorders associated with the puerperium should be coded according to the presenting psychiatric disorder, while a second code from ICD-10 (O99.3) will indicate the association with the puerperium.

F53.0 Mild mental and behavioural disorders associated with the puerperium, not elsewhere classified

F53.1 Severe mental and behavioural disorders associated with the puerperium, not elsewhere classified

F53.8 Other mental and behavioural disorders associated with the puerperium, not elsewhere classified

F53.9 Puerperal mental disorder, unspecified

F54 Psychological and behavioural factors associated with disorders or diseases classified elsewhere

This category should be used to record the presence of psychological or behavioural factors thought to have influenced the manifestation, or affected the course, of physical disorders that can be classified using other chapters of ICD-10. Any resulting mental disturbances are usually mild and often prolonged (such as worry, emotional conflict, apprehension) and do not of themselves justify the use of any of the categories described in the rest of this book. An additional code should be used to identify the physical disorder. (In the rare instances in which an overt psychiatric disorder is thought to have caused a physical disorder, a second additional code should be used to record the psychiatric disorder.)

F55 Abuse of non-dependence-producing substances

A wide variety of medicaments and folk remedies may be involved, but the particularly important groups are: psychotropic drugs that do not produce dependence, such as antidepressants; laxatives; and analgesics that may be purchased without medical prescription, such as aspirin and paracetamol. Although the medication may have been medically prescribed or recommended in the first instance, prolonged, unnecessary, and often excessive dosage develops, which is facilitated by the availability of the substances without medical prescription.

Persistent and unjustified use of these substances is usually associated with unnecessary expense, often involves unnecessary contacts with medical professionals or supporting staff, and is sometimes marked by the harmful physical effects of the substances. Attempts to discourage or forbid the use of the substance are often met with resistance; for laxatives and analgesics this may be in spite of warnings about (or even the development of) physical harm such as renal dysfunction or electrolyte disturbances. Although it is usually clear that the patient has a strong motivation to take the substance, no dependence or withdrawal symptoms develop as in the case of the psychoactive substances specified in F10–F19.

A fourth character may be used to identify the type of substance involved:

F55.0 Antidepressants

(such as tricyclic and tetracyclic antidepressants and monoamine oxidase inhibitors)

F55.1 Laxatives

F55.2 Analgesics

(such as aspirin, paracetamol, phenacetin, not specified as psychoactive in F10–F19)

F55.3 Antacids

F55.4 Vitamins

F55.5 Steroids or hormones

F55.6 Specific herbal or folk remedies

F55.8 Other substances that do not produce dependence

(such as diuretics)

F55.9 Unspecified

F59 Unspecified behavioural syndromes associated with physiological disturbances and physical factors

F60 – F69
Disorders of adult personality and behaviour

F60 Specific personality disorders

G1. There is evidence that the individual's characteristic and enduring patterns of inner experience and behaviour as a whole deviate markedly from the culturally expected and accepted range (or "norm"). Such deviation must be manifest in more than one of the following areas:

(1) cognition (i.e. ways of perceiving and interpreting things, people, and events; forming attitudes and images of self and others);

(2) affectivity (range, intensity, and appropriateness of emotional arousal and response);

(3) control over impulses and gratification of needs;

(4) manner of relating to others and of handling interpersonal situations.

G2. The deviation must manifest itself pervasively as behaviour that is inflexible, maladaptive, or otherwise dysfunctional across a broad range of personal and social situations (i.e. not being limited to one specific "triggering" stimulus or situation).

G3. There is personal distress, or adverse impact on the social environment, or both, clearly attributable to the behaviour referred to in criterion G2.

G4. There must be evidence that the deviation is stable and of long duration, having its onset in late childhood or adolescence.

G5. The deviation cannot be explained as a manifestation or consequence of other adult mental disorders, although episodic or chronic conditions from sections F00–F59 or F70–F79 of this classification may coexist with, or be superimposed upon, the deviation.

G6. Organic brain disease, injury, or dysfunction must be excluded as the possible cause of the deviation. (If an organic causation is demonstrable, category F07.- should be used.)

Comments

The assessment of criteria G1–G6 above should be based on as many sources of information as possible. Although it is sometimes possible to obtain sufficient evidence from a single interview with the individual, as a general rule it is recommended to have more than one interview with the person and to collect history data from informants or past records.

It is suggested that sub-criteria should be developed to define behaviour patterns specific to different cultural settings concerning social norms, rules, and obligations where needed (such as examples of irresponsibility and disregard of social norms in dissocial personality disorder).

The diagnosis of personality disorder for research purposes requires the identification of a subtype. (More than one subtype can be coded if there is compelling evidence that the individual meets multiple sets of criteria.)

F60.0 Paranoid personality disorder

A. The general criteria for personality disorder (F60) must be met.

B. At least four of the following must be present:

(1) excessive sensitivity to setbacks and rebuffs;

(2) tendency to bear grudges persistently, e.g. refusal to forgive insults, injuries, or slights;

(3) suspiciousness and a pervasive tendency to distort experience by misconstruing the neutral or friendly actions of others as hostile or contemptuous;

(4) a combative and tenacious sense of personal rights out of keeping with the actual situation;

(5) recurrent suspicions, without justification, regarding sexual fidelity of spouse or sexual partner;

(6) persistent self-referential attitude, associated particularly with excessive self-importance;

(7) preoccupation with unsubstantiated "conspiratorial" explanations of events either immediate to the patient or in the world at large.

F60.1 Schizoid personality disorder

A. The general criteria for personality disorder (F60) must be met.

B. At least four of the following must be present:

(1) few, if any, activities provide pleasure;

(2) display of emotional coldness, detachment, or flattened affectivity;

(3) limited capacity to express either warm, tender feelings or anger towards others;

(4) an appearance of indifference to either praise or criticism;

(5) little interest in having sexual experiences with another person (taking into account age);

(6) consistent choice of solitary activities;

(7) excessive preoccupation with fantasy and introspection;

(8) no desire for, or possession of, any close friends or confiding relationships (or only one);

(9) marked insensitivity to prevailing social norms and conventions; disregard for such norms and conventions is unintentional.

F60.2 Dissocial personality disorder

A. The general criteria for personality disorder (F60) must be met.

B. At least three of the following must be present:

(1) callous unconcern for the feelings of others;

(2) gross and persistent attitude of irresponsibility and disregard for social norms, rules, and obligations;

(3) incapacity to maintain enduring relationships, though with no difficulty in establishing them;

(4) very low tolerance to frustration and a low threshold for discharge of aggression, including violence;

(5) incapacity to experience guilt, or to profit from adverse experience, particularly punishment;

(6) marked proneness to blame others, or to offer plausible rationalizations for the behaviour that has brought the individual into conflict with society.

Comments

Persistent irritability and the presence of conduct disorder during childhood and adolescence complete the clinical picture but are not required for the diagnosis.

It is suggested that sub-criteria should be developed to define behaviour patterns specific to different cultural settings concerning social norms, rules, and obligations where needed (such as examples of irresponsibility and disregard of social norms).

F60.3 Emotionally unstable personality disorder

F60.30 Impulsive type

A. The general criteria for personality disorder (F60) must be met.

B. At least three of the following must be present, one of which must be (2):

(1) marked tendency to act unexpectedly and without consideration of the consequences;

(2) marked tendency to quarrelsome behaviour and to conflicts with others, especially when impulsive acts are thwarted or criticized;

(3) liability to outbursts of anger or violence, with inability to control the resulting behavioural explosions;

(4) difficulty in maintaining any course of action that offers no immediate reward;

(5) unstable and capricious mood.

F60.31 Borderline type

A. The general criteria for personality disorder (F60) must be met.

B. At least three of the symptoms mentioned in criterion B for F60.30 must be present, with at least two of the following in addition:

(1) disturbances in and uncertainty about self-image, aims, and internal preferences (including sexual);

(2) liability to become involved in intense and unstable relationships, often leading to emotional crises;

(3) excessive efforts to avoid abandonment;

(4) recurrent threats or acts of self-harm;
(5) chronic feelings of emptiness.

F60.4 Histrionic personality disorder

A. The general criteria for personality disorder (F60) must be met.

B. At least four of the following must be present:
(1) self-dramatization, theatricality, or exaggerated expression of emotions;
(2) suggestibility (the individual is easily influenced by others or by circumstances);
(3) shallow and labile affectivity;
(4) continual seeking for excitement and activities in which the individual is the centre of attention;
(5) inappropriate seductiveness in appearance or behaviour;
(6) over-concern with physical attractiveness.

Comments

Egocentricity, self-indulgence, continuous longing for appreciation, lack of consideration for others, feelings that are easily hurt, and persistent manipulative behaviour complete the clinical picture, but are not required for the diagnosis.

F60.5 Anankastic personality disorder

Note. This disorder is often referred to as obsessive–compulsive personality disorder.

A. The general criteria for personality disorder (F60) must be met.

B. At least four of the following must be present:
(1) feelings of excessive doubt and caution;
(2) preoccupation with details, rules, lists, order, organization, or schedule;
(3) perfectionism that interferes with task completion;
(4) excessive conscientiousness and scrupulousness;
(5) undue preoccupation with productivity to the exclusion of pleasure and interpersonal relationships;
(6) excessive pedantry and adherence to social conventions;
(7) rigidity and stubbornness;

(8) unreasonable insistence by the individual that others submit to exactly his or her way of doing things, or unreasonable reluctance to allow others to do things.

F60.6 Anxious [avoidant] personality disorder

A. The general criteria for personality disorder (F60) must be met.

B. At least four of the following must be present:

(1) persistent and pervasive feelings of tension and apprehension;

(2) belief that one is socially inept, personally unappealing, or inferior to others;

(3) excessive preoccupation with being criticized or rejected in social situations;

(4) unwillingness to become involved with people unless certain of being liked;

(5) restrictions in lifestyle because of need for physical security;

(6) avoidance of social or occupational activities that involve significant interpersonal contact, because of fear of criticism, disapproval, or rejection.

F60.7 Dependent personality disorder

A. The general criteria for personality disorder (F60) must be met.

B. At least four of the following must be present:

(1) encouraging or allowing others to make most of one's important life decisions;

(2) subordination of one's own needs to those of others on whom one is dependent, and undue compliance with their wishes;

(3) unwillingness to make even reasonable demands on the people one depends on;

(4) feeling uncomfortable or helpless when alone, because of exaggerated fears of inability to care for oneself;

(5) preoccupation with fears of being left to care for oneself;

(6) limited capacity to make everyday decisions without an excessive amount of advice and reassurance from others.

F60.8 Other specific personality disorders

If none of the preceding rubrics is fitting, but a condition meeting the general criteria for personality disorder listed under F60 is nevertheless present, this code should be used (see also Annex 1). An extra character may be added for identifying specific personality disorders not currently in ICD-10. In using code F60.8, it is recommended always to record a vignette description of the specific disorder.

F60.9 Personality disorder, unspecified

F61 Mixed and other personality disorders

No attempt has been made to provide standard sets of criteria for these mixed disorders, since those doing research in this field will prefer to state their own criteria depending upon the purpose of their studies.

F61.0[1] Mixed personality disorders

Features of several of the disorders in F60.– are present, but not to the extent that the criteria for any of the specified personality disorders in that category are met.

F61.1[1] Troublesome personality changes

Not classifiable in F60.– or F62.– and regarded as secondary to a main diagnosis of a coexisting affective or anxiety disorder.

F62 Enduring personality changes, not attributable to brain damage and disease

F62.0 Enduring personality change after catastrophic experience

A. There must be evidence (from the personal history or from key informants) of a definite and persistent change in the individual's pattern of perceiving, relating to, and thinking about the environment and the self, following exposure to catastrophic stress (e.g. concentration camp experience; torture; disaster; prolonged exposure to life-threatening situations).

B. The personality change should be significant and represent inflexible and maladaptive features as indicated by the presence of at least two of the following:

(1) a permanent hostile or distrustful attitude towards the world in a person who previously showed no such traits;

[1] This four-character code is not included in Chapter V(F) of ICD-10.

(2) social withdrawal (avoidance of contacts with people other than a few close relatives with whom the individual lives) which is not due to another current mental disorder (such as a mood disorder);

(3) a constant feeling of emptiness or hopelessness, not limited to a discrete episode of mood disorder, which was not present before the catastrophic stress experience; this may be associated with increased dependency on others, inability to express negative or aggressive feelings, and prolonged depressive mood without any evidence of depressive disorder before exposure to the catastrophic stress;

(4) an enduring feeling of being "on edge" or of being threatened without any external cause, as evidenced by an increased vigilance and irritability in a person who previously showed no such traits or hyper-alertness; this chronic state of inner tension and feeling threatened may be associated with a tendency to excessive drinking or use of drugs;

(5) a permanent feeling of being changed or of being different from others (estrangement); this feeling may be associated with an experience of emotional numbness.

C. The change should cause significant interference with personal functioning in daily living, personal distress, or adverse impact on the social environment.

D. The personality change should have developed after the catastrophic experience, and there should be no history of a pre-existing adult personality disorder or trait accentuation, or of personality or developmental disorders during childhood or adolescence, that could explain the current personality traits.

E. The personality change must have been present for at least 2 years. It is not related to episodes of any other mental disorder (except post-traumatic stress disorder) and cannot be explained by brain damage or disease.

F. The personality change meeting the above criteria is often preceded by a post-traumatic stress disorder (F43.1). The symptoms of the two conditions can overlap and the personality change may be a chronic outcome of a post-traumatic stress disorder. However, an enduring personality change should not be assumed in such cases unless, in addition to at least 2 years of post-traumatic stress disorder, there has been a further period of no less than 2 years during which the above criteria have been met.

F62.1 Enduring personality change after psychiatric illness

A. There must be evidence of a definite and enduring change in the individual's pattern of perceiving, relating to, and thinking about the environment and the self, following the experience of suffering from one or several episodes of psychiatric illness from which he or she has recovered clinically without residual symptoms.

B. The personality change should be significant and represent inflexible and maladaptive features as indicated by the presence of at least two of the following:

(1) dependence on others (the individual passively assumes, or demands, that others take responsibility for his or her own life, and is unwilling to decide on important issues related to his or her actions or future);

(2) social withdrawal or isolation, which is secondary to a conviction (not delusional) or feeling of being "changed" or stigmatized as a result of the illness; this conviction or feeling may be strengthened by societal attitudes but cannot be completely explained by the objective social circumstances; feeling vulnerable to others' moral opprobrium (narcissistic injury) may also be a factor but such feeling should be egosyntonic if it is to be considered an enduring personality trait;

(3) passivity, reduced interests, and diminished involvement in previously entertained leisure activities (which may reinforce the social isolation);

(4) a change in self-perception, leading to a frequent or constant claim of being ill; this may be associated with hypochondriacal behaviour and an increased utilization of psychiatric or other medical services;

(5) a demanding attitude towards other people in which the individual expects special favours or considers himself or herself deserving of special attention or treatment;

(6) dysphoric or labile mood, not due to a current mental disorder or antecedent mental disorder with residual affective symptoms.

C. The personality change following the psychiatric illness must be understandable in terms of the individual's subjective emotional experience of the situation, his or her previous adjustment, vulnerabilities, and life-situation including the attitudes or reactions of significant others following the illness.

D. The personality change should cause significant interference with personal functioning in daily living, personal distress, or adverse impact on the social environment.

E. There should be no history of a pre-existing adult personality disorder or trait accentuation or of personality or developmental disorders during childhood or adolescence that could explain the current personality traits.

F. The personality change has been present for at least 2 years and is not a manifestation of another mental disorder or secondary to brain damage or disease.

F62.8 Other enduring personality changes

F62.9 Enduring personality change, unspecified

F63 Habit and impulse disorders

F63.0 Pathological gambling

A. Two or more episodes of gambling occur over a period of at least 1 year.

B. These episodes do not have a profitable outcome for the individual, but are continued despite personal distress and interference with personal functioning in daily living.

C. The individual describes an intense urge to gamble which is difficult to control, and reports that he or she is unable to stop gambling by an effort of will.

D. The individual is preoccupied with thoughts or mental images of the act of gambling or the circumstances surrounding the act.

F63.1 Pathological fire-setting [pyromania]

A. There are two or more acts of fire-setting without apparent motive.

B. The individual describes an intense urge to set fire to objects, with a feeling of tension before the act and relief afterwards.

C. The individual is preoccupied with thoughts or mental images of fire-setting or of the circumstances surrounding the act (e.g. abnormal interest in fire-engines or in calling out the fire service).

F63.2 Pathological stealing [kleptomania]

A. There are two or more thefts in which the individual steals without any apparent motive of personal gain or gain for another person.

B. The individual describes an intense urge to steal, with a feeling of tension before the act and relief afterwards.

F63.3 Trichotillomania

A. Noticeable hair-loss is caused by the individual's persistent and recurrent failure to resist impulses to pull out hairs.

B. The individual describes an intense urge to pull out hairs, with mounting tension before the act and a sense of relief afterwards.

C. There is no pre-existing inflammation of the skin, and the hair-pulling is not in response to a delusion or hallucination.

F63.8 Other habit and impulse disorders

This category should be used for other kinds of persistently repeated maladaptive behaviour that are not secondary to a recognized psychiatric syndrome, and in which it appears that there is repeated failure to resist impulses to carry out the behaviour. There is a prodromal period of tension with a feeling of release at the time of the act.

F63.9 Habit and impulse disorder, unspecified

F64 Gender identity disorders

F64.0 Transsexualism

A. The individual desires to live and be accepted as a member of the opposite sex, usually accompanied by the wish to make his or her body as congruent as possible with the preferred sex through surgery and hormonal treatment.

B. The transsexual identity has been present persistently for at least 2 years.

C. The disorder is not a symptom of another mental disorder, such as schizophrenia, nor is it associated with chromosome abnormality.

F64.1 Dual-role transvestism

A. The individual wears clothes of the opposite sex in order to experience temporarily membership of the opposite sex.

B. There is no sexual motivation for the cross-dressing.

C. The individual has no desire for a permanent change to the opposite sex.

F64.2 Gender identity disorder of childhood

For girls:

A. The individual shows persistent and intense distress about being a girl, and has a stated desire to be a boy (not merely a desire for any perceived cultural advantages to being a boy), or insists that she is a boy.

B. Either of the following must be present:

(1) persistent marked aversion to normative feminine clothing and insistence on wearing stereotypical masculine clothing, e.g. boys' underwear and other accessories;

(2) persistent repudiation of female anatomical structures, as evidenced by at least one of the following:

(a) an assertion that she has, or will grow, a penis;
(b) rejection of urinating in a sitting position;
(c) assertion that she does not want to grow breasts or menstruate.

C. The girl has not yet reached puberty.

D. The disorder must have been present for at least 6 months.

For boys:

A. The individual shows persistent and intense distress about being a boy, and has an intense desire to be a girl or, more rarely, insists that he is a girl.

B. Either of the following must be present:

(1) preoccupation with stereotypical female activities, as shown by a preference for either cross-dressing or simulating female attire, or by an intense desire to participate in the games and pastimes of girls and rejection of stereotypical male toys, games, and activities;

(2) persistent repudiation of male anatomical structures, as indicated by at least one of the following repeated assertions:

(a) that he will grow up to become a woman (not merely in role);
(b) that his penis or testes are disgusting or will disappear;
(c) that it would be better not to have a penis or testes.

C. The boy has not yet reached puberty.

D. The disorder must have been present for at least 6 months.

F64.8 Other gender identity disorders

F64.9 Gender identity disorder, unspecified

F65 Disorders of sexual preference

G1. The individual experiences recurrent intense sexual urges and fantasies involving unusual objects or activities.

G2. The individual either acts on the urges or is markedly distressed by them.

G3. The preference has been present for at least 6 months.

F65.0 Fetishism

A. The general criteria for disorders of sexual preference (F65) must be met.

B. The fetish (some non-living object) is the most important source of sexual stimulation or is essential for satisfactory sexual response.

F65.1 Fetishistic transvestism

A. The general criteria for disorders of sexual preference (F65) must be met.

B. The individual wears articles of clothing of the opposite sex in order to create the appearance and feeling of being a member of the opposite sex.

C. The cross-dressing is closely associated with sexual arousal. Once orgasm occurs and sexual arousal declines, there is a strong desire to remove the clothing.

F65.2 Exhibitionism

A. The general criteria for disorders of sexual preference (F65) must be met.

B. There is either a recurrent or a persistent tendency to expose the genitalia to unsuspecting strangers (usually of the opposite sex), which is almost invariably associated with sexual arousal and masturbation.

C. There is no intention or invitation to have sexual intercourse with the "witness(es)".

F65.3 Voyeurism

A. The general criteria for disorders of sexual preference (F65) must be met.

B. There is either a recurrent or a persistent tendency to look at people engaging in sexual or intimate behaviour such as undressing, which is associated with sexual excitement and masturbation.

C. There is no intention to reveal one's presence.

D. There is no intention of sexual involvement with the person(s) observed.

F65.4 Paedophilia

A. The general criteria for disorders of sexual preference (F65) must be met.

B. There is a persistent or predominant preference for sexual activity with a prepubescent child or children.

C. The individual is at least 16 years old and at least 5 years older than the child or children in criterion B.

F65.5 Sadomasochism

A. The general criteria for disorders of sexual preference (F65) must be met.

B. There is preference for sexual activity, as recipient (masochism) or provider (sadism), or both, which involves at least one of the following:

(1) pain;
(2) humiliation;
(3) bondage.

C. The sadomasochistic activity is the most important source of stimulation or is necessary for sexual gratification.

F65.6 Multiple disorders of sexual preference

The likelihood of more than one abnormal sexual preference occurring in one individual is greater than would be expected by chance. For research purposes the different types of preference, and their relative importance to the individual, should be listed. The most common combination is fetishism, transvestism, and sadomasochism.

F65.8 Other disorders of sexual preference

A variety of other patterns of sexual preference and activity may occur, each being relatively uncommon. These include such activities as making obscene telephone calls, rubbing up against people for sexual stimulation in crowded public places (frotteurism), sexual activity with animals, use of strangulation or anoxia for intensifying sexual excitement, and a preference for partners with some particular anatomical abnormality such as an amputated limb.

Erotic practices are too diverse and many too rare or idiosyncratic to justify a separate term for each. Swallowing urine, smearing faeces, or piercing foreskin or nipples may be part of the behavioural repertoire in sadomasochism. Masturbatory rituals of various kinds are common, but the more extreme practices, such as the insertion of objects into the rectum or penile urethra, or partial self-strangulation, when they take the place of ordinary sexual contacts, amount to abnormalities. Necrophilia should also be coded here.

F65.9 Disorder of sexual preference, unspecified

F66 Psychological and behavioural disorders associated with sexual development and orientation

This section is intended to cover those types of problem that derive from variations of sexual development or orientation, when the sexual preference *per se* is not necessarily problematic or abnormal.

F66.0 Sexual maturation disorder

The patient suffers from uncertainty about his or her gender identity or sexual orientation, which causes anxiety or depression.

F66.1 Egodystonic sexual orientation

The gender identity or sexual preference is not in doubt, but the individual wishes it were different.

F66.2 Sexual relationship disorder

The abnormality of gender identity or sexual preference is responsible for difficulties in forming or maintaining a relationship with a sexual partner.

F66.8 Other psychosexual development disorders

F66.9 Psychosexual development disorder, unspecified

F68 Other disorders of adult personality and behaviour

F68.0 Elaboration of physical symptoms for psychological reasons

A. Physical symptoms originally due to a confirmed physical disorder, disease, or disability become exaggerated or prolonged in excess of what can be explained by the physical disorder itself.

B. There is evidence for a psychological causation for the excess symptoms (such as evident fear of disability or death, possible financial compensation, disappointment at the standard of care experienced).

F68.1 Intentional production or feigning of symptoms or disabilities, either physical or psychological [factitious disorder]

A. The individual exhibits a persistent pattern of intentional production or feigning of symptoms and/or self-infliction of wounds in order to produce symptoms.

B. No evidence can be found for an external motivation such as financial compensation, escape from danger, or more medical care. (If such evidence can be found, category Z76.5, malingering, should be used.)

C. *Most commonly used exclusion clause.* There is no confirmed physical or mental disorder that could explain the symptoms.

F68.8 Other specified disorders of adult personality and behaviour

This category should be used for coding any specified disorder of adult personality and behaviour that cannot be classified under any one of the preceding headings.

F69 Unspecified disorder of adult personality and behaviour

This code should be used only as a last resort, if the presence of a disorder of adult personality and behaviour can be assumed, but information to allow its diagnosis and allocation to a specific category is lacking.

F70 – F79
Mental retardation

Detailed clinical diagnostic criteria that can be used internationally for research cannot be specified for mental retardation in the same way as they can for most of the other disorders in Chapter V(F) of ICD-10. This is because manifestations of the two main components of mental retardation, namely low cognitive ability and diminished social competence, are profoundly affected by social and cultural influences. Only general guidance can be given here about the most appropriate methods of assessment to use.

Level of cognitive abilities

Depending upon the cultural norms and expectations of the individuals being studied, research workers must make their own judgements as to how best to estimate intelligence quotient (IQ) or mental age according to the bands given below:

Category	*Mental retardation*	*IQ range*	*Mental age (years)*
F70	Mild	50–69	9 to under 12
F71	Moderate	35–49	6 to under 9
F72	Severe	20–34	3 to under 6
F73	Profound	Below 20	Less than 3

Level of social competence

Within most European and north American cultures, the Vineland Social Maturity Scale[1] is recommended for use, if it is judged to be appropriate. Modified versions or equivalent scales should be developed for use in other cultures.

A fourth character may be used to specify the extent of associated impairment of behaviour:

F7*x*.0 No, or minimal, impairment of behaviour

F7*x*.1 Significant impairment of behaviour requiring attention or treatment

F7*x*.8 Other impairments of behaviour

F7*x*.9 Without mention of impairment of behaviour

---

[1] Doll EA. *Vineland Social Maturity Scale, condensed manual of directions.* Circle Pines MN, American Guidance Service Inc., 1965.

Comments

A specially designed multi-axial system is required to do justice to the variety of personal, clinical, and social statements needed for the comprehensive assessment of the causes and consequences of mental retardation. One such system is now in preparation for this section of Chapter V(F) of ICD-10.

F80 – F89
Disorders of psychological development

F80 Specific developmental disorders of speech and language

F80.0 Specific speech articulation disorder

Note. This disorder is also referred to as specific speech phonological disorder.

A. Articulation (phonological) skills, as assessed on standardized tests, are below the 2 standard deviations limit for the child's age.

B. Articulation (phonological) skills are at least 1 standard deviation below non-verbal IQ as assessed on standardized tests.

C. Language expression and comprehension, as assessed on standardized tests, are within the 2 standard deviations limit for the child's age.

D. There are no neurological, sensory, or physical impairments that directly affect speech sound production, nor is there a pervasive developmental disorder (F84.–).

E. *Most commonly used exclusion clause.* Non-verbal IQ is below 70 on a standardized test.

F80.1 Expressive language disorder

A. Expressive language skills, as assessed on standardized tests, are below the 2 standard deviations limit for the child's age.

B. Expressive language skills are at least 1 standard deviation below non-verbal IQ as assessed on standardized tests.

C. Receptive language skills, as assessed on standardized tests, are within the 2 standard deviations limit for the child's age.

D. Use and understanding of non-verbal communication and imaginative language functions are within the normal range.

E. There are no neurological, sensory, or physical impairments that directly affect use of spoken language, nor is there a pervasive developmental disorder (F84.–).

F. *Most commonly used exclusion clause.* Non-verbal IQ is below 70 on a standardized test.

F80.2 Receptive language disorder

Note. This disorder is also referred to as mixed receptive/expressive disorder.

A. Language comprehension, as assessed on standardized tests, is below the 2 standard deviations limit for the child's age.

B. Receptive language skills are at least 1 standard deviation below non-verbal IQ as assessed on standardized tests.

C. There are no neurological, sensory, or physical impairments that directly affect receptive language, nor is there a pervasive developmental disorder (F84.–).

D. *Most commonly used exclusion clause.* Non-verbal IQ is below 70 on a standardized test.

F80.3 Acquired aphasia with epilepsy [Landau–Kleffner syndrome]

A. Severe loss of expressive and receptive language skills occurs over a period of time not exceeding 6 months.

B. Language development was normal before the loss.

C. Paroxysmal EEG abnormalities affecting one or both temporal lobes become apparent within a time span extending from 2 years before to 2 years after the initial loss of language.

D. Hearing is within the normal range.

E. A level of non-verbal intelligence within the normal range is retained.

F. There is no diagnosable neurological condition other than that implicit in the abnormal EEG and presence of epileptic seizures (when they occur).

G. The disorder does not meet the criteria for a pervasive developmental disorder (F84.–).

F80.8 Other developmental disorders of speech and language

F80.9 Developmental disorder of speech and language, unspecified

This category should be avoided as far as possible and should be used only for unspecified disorders in which there is significant impairment in the development of speech or language that cannot be accounted for by mental retardation, or by neurological, sensory, or physical impairments that directly affect speech or language.

F81 Specific developmental disorders of scholastic skills

F81.0 Specific reading disorder

A. Either of the following must be present:

(1) a score on reading accuracy and/or comprehension that is at least 2 standard errors of prediction below the level expected on the basis of the child's chronological age and general intelligence, with both reading skills and IQ assessed on an individually administered test standardized for the child's culture and educational system;

(2) a history of serious reading difficulties, or test scores that met criterion A(1) at an earlier age, plus a score on a spelling test that is at least 2 standard errors of prediction below the level expected on the basis of the child's chronological age and IQ.

B. The disturbance described in criterion A significantly interferes with academic achievement or with activities of daily living that require reading skills.

C. The disorder is not the direct result of a defect in visual or hearing acuity, or of a neurological disorder.

D. School experiences are within the average expectable range (i.e. there have been no extreme inadequacies in educational experiences).

E. *Most commonly used exclusion clause.* IQ is below 70 on an individually administered standardized test.

Possible additional inclusion criterion

For some research purposes, investigators may wish to specify a history of some level of impairment during the preschool years in speech, language, sound categorization, motor coordination, visual processing, attention, or control or modulation of activity.

Comments

The above criteria would not include general reading backwardness of a type that would fall within the clinical guidelines. The research diagnostic criteria for general reading backwardness would be the same as for specific reading disorder except that criterion A(1) would specify reading skills 2 standard errors of prediction below the level expected on the basis of chronological age (i.e. not taking IQ into account), and criterion A(2) would follow the same principle for spelling. The validity of the differentiation between these two varieties of reading problem is not unequivocally established, but it seems that the specific type has a more specific association with language retardation (whereas general reading backwardness is associated with a wider range of developmental disabilities), and is more prevalent in boys than in girls.

There are further research differentiations that are based on analyses of the types of spelling error.

F81.1 Specific spelling disorder

A. The score on a standardized spelling test is at least 2 standard errors of prediction below the level expected on the basis of the child's chronological age and general intelligence.

B. Scores on reading accuracy and comprehension and on arithmetic are within the normal range (± 2 standard deviations from the mean).

C. There is no history of significant reading difficulties.

D. School experience is within the average expectable range (i.e. there have been no extreme inadequacies in educational experiences).

E. Spelling difficulties have been present from the early stages of learning to spell.

F. The disturbance described in criterion A significantly interferes with academic achievement or with activities of daily living that require spelling skills.

G. *Most commonly used exclusion clause.* IQ is below 70 on an individually administered standardized test.

F81.2 Specific disorder of arithmetical skills

A. The score on a standardized arithmetic test is at least 2 standard errors of prediction below the level expected on the basis of the child's chronological age and general intelligence.

B. Scores on reading accuracy and comprehension and on spelling are within the normal range (± 2 standard deviations from the mean).

C. There is no history of significant reading or spelling difficulties.

D. School experience is within the average expectable range (i.e. there have been no extreme inadequacies in educational experiences).

E. Arithmetical difficulties have been present from the early stages of learning arithmetic.

F. The disturbance described in criterion A significantly interferes with academic achievement or with activities of daily living that require arithmetical skills.

G. *Most commonly used exclusion clause.* IQ is below 70 on an individually administered standardized test.

F81.3 Mixed disorder of scholastic skills

This is an ill-defined, inadequately conceptualized (but necessary) residual category of disorders in which both arithmetical and reading or spelling skills are significantly impaired, but in which the disorder is not solely explicable in terms of general mental retardation or inadequate schooling. It should be used for disorders meeting the criteria for F81.2 and either F81.0 or F81.1.

F81.8 Other developmental disorders of scholastic skills

F81.9 Developmental disorder of scholastic skills, unspecified

This category should be avoided as far as possible and should be used only for unspecified disorders in which there is a significant disability of learning that cannot be solely accounted for by mental retardation, visual acuity problems, or inadequate schooling.

F82 Specific developmental disorder of motor function

A. The score on a standardized test of fine or gross motor coordination is at least 2 standard deviations below the level expected for the child's chronological age.

B. The disturbance described in criterion A significantly interferes with academic achievement or with activities of daily living.

C. There is no diagnosable neurological disorder.

D. *Most commonly used exclusion clause.* IQ is below 70 on an individually administered standardized test.

F83 Mixed specific developmental disorders

This is an ill-defined, inadequately conceptualized (but necessary) residual category of disorders in which there is some admixture of specific developmental disorders of speech and language, of scholastic skills, or of motor function, but in which none predominates sufficiently to constitute the prime diagnosis. It is common for each of these specific developmental disorders to be associated with some degree of general impairment of cognitive functions, and this mixed category should be used only when there is a major overlap. Thus, the category should be used when there are dysfunctions meeting the criteria for two or more of F80.–, F81.–, and F82.

F84 Pervasive developmental disorders

F84.0 Childhood autism

A. Abnormal or impaired development is evident before the age of 3 years in at least one of the following areas:

(1) receptive or expressive language as used in social communication;

(2) the development of selective social attachments or of reciprocal social interaction;

(3) functional or symbolic play.

B. A total of at least six symptoms from (1), (2), and (3) must be present, with at least two from (1) and at least one from each of (2) and (3):

(1) Qualitative abnormalities in reciprocal social interaction are manifest in at least two of the following areas:

(a) failure adequately to use eye-to-eye gaze, facial expression, body posture, and gesture to regulate social interaction;

(b) failure to develop (in a manner appropriate to mental age, and despite ample opportunities) peer relationships that involve a mutual sharing of interests, activities, and emotions;

(c) lack of socio-emotional reciprocity as shown by an impaired or deviant response to other people's emotions; or lack of modulation of behaviour according to social context; or a weak integration of social, emotional, and communicative behaviours;

(d) lack of spontaneous seeking to share enjoyment, interests, or achievements with other people (e.g. a lack of showing, bringing, or pointing out to other people objects of interest to the individual).

(2) Qualitative abnormalities in communication are manifest in at least one of the following areas:

(a) a delay in, or total lack of, development of spoken language that is *not* accompanied by an attempt to compensate through the use of gesture or mime as an alternative mode of communication (often preceded by a lack of communicative babbling);

(b) relative failure to initiate or sustain conversational interchange (at whatever level of language skills is present), in which there is reciprocal responsiveness to the communications of the other person;

(c) stereotyped and repetitive use of language or idiosyncratic use of words or phrases;

(d) lack of varied spontaneous make-believe or (when young) social imitative play.

(3) Restricted, repetitive, and stereotyped patterns of behaviour, interests, and activities are manifest in at least one of the following areas:

(a) an encompassing preoccupation with one or more stereotyped and restricted patterns of interest that are abnormal in content or focus; or one or more interests that are abnormal in their intensity and circumscribed nature though not in their content or focus;

(b) apparently compulsive adherence to specific, non-functional routines or rituals;

(c) stereotyped and repetitive motor mannerisms that involve either hand or finger flapping or twisting, or complex whole body movements;

(d) preoccupations with part-objects or non-functional elements of play materials (such as their odour, the feel of their surface, or the noise or vibration that they generate).

C. The clinical picture is not attributable to the other varieties of pervasive developmental disorder: specific developmental disorder of receptive language (F80.2) with secondary socio-emotional problems; reactive attachment disorder (F94.1) or disinhibited attachment disorder (F94.2); mental retardation (F70–F72) with some associated emotional or behavioural disorder; schizophrenia (F20.–) of unusually early onset; and Rett's syndrome (F84.2).

F84.1 Atypical autism

A. Abnormal or impaired development is evident at or after the age of 3 years (criteria as for autism except for age of manifestation).

B. There are qualitative abnormalities in reciprocal social interaction or in communication, or restricted, repetitive, and stereotyped patterns of behaviour, interests, and activities. (Criteria as for autism except that it is unnecessary to meet the criteria for number of areas of abnormality.)

C. The disorder does not meet the diagnostic criteria for autism (F84.0).

Autism may be atypical in either age of onset (F84.10) or symptomatology (F84.11); the two types are differentiated with a fifth character for research purposes. Syndromes that are atypical in both respects should be coded F84.12.

F84.10 Atypicality in age of onset

A. The disorder does not meet criterion A for autism (F84.0); that is, abnormal or impaired development is evident only at or after the age of 3 years.

B. The disorder meets criteria B and C for autism (F84.0).

F84.11 Atypicality in symptomatology

A. The disorder meets criterion A for autism (F84.0); that is abnormal or impaired development is evident before the age of 3 years.

B. There are qualitative abnormalities in reciprocal social interactions or in communication, or restricted, repetitive, and stereotyped patterns of behaviour, interests, and activities. (Criteria as for autism except that it is unnecessary to meet the criteria for number of areas of abnormality.)

C. The disorder meets criterion C for autism (F84.0).

D. The disorder does not fully meet criterion B for autism (F84.0).

F84.12 Atypicality in both age of onset and symptomatology

A. The disorder does not meet criterion A for autism (F84.0); that is, abnormal or impaired development is evident only at or after the age of 3 years.

B. There are qualitative abnormalities in reciprocal social interactions or in communication, or restricted, repetitive, and stereotyped patterns of behaviour, interests, and activities. (Criteria as for autism except that it is unnecessary to meet the criteria for number of areas of abnormality.)

C. The disorder meets criterion C for autism (F84.0).

D. The disorder does not fully meet criterion B for autism (F84.0).

F84.2 Rett's syndrome

A. There is an apparently normal prenatal and perinatal period *and* apparently normal psychomotor development through the first 5 months *and* normal head circumference at birth.

B. There is deceleration of head growth between 5 months and 4 years *and* loss of acquired purposeful hand skills between 5 and 30 months of age that is associated with concurrent communication dysfunction and impaired social interactions *and* the appearance of poorly coordinated/unstable gait and/or trunk movements.

C. There is severe impairment of expressive and receptive language, together with severe psychomotor retardation.

D. There are stereotyped midline hand movements (such as hand-wringing or "hand-washing") with an onset at or after the time when purposeful hand movements are lost.

F84.3 Other childhood disintegrative disorder

A. Development is apparently normal up to the age of at least 2 years. The presence of normal age-appropriate skills in communication, social relationships, play, and adaptive behaviour at age 2 years or later is required for diagnosis.

B. There is a definite loss of previously acquired skills at about the time of onset of the disorder. The diagnosis requires a clinically significant loss of skills (not just a failure to use them in certain situations) in at least two of the following areas:

(1) expressive or receptive language;

(2) play;

(3) social skills or adaptive behaviour;

(4) bowel or bladder control;

(5) motor skills.

C. Qualitatively abnormal social functioning is manifest in at least two of the following areas:

(1) qualitative abnormalities in reciprocal social interaction (of the type defined for autism);

(2) qualitative abnormalities in communication (of the type defined for autism);

(3) restricted, repetitive, and stereotyped patterns of behaviour, interests, and activities, including motor stereotypies and mannerisms;

(4) a general loss of interest in objects and in the environment.

D. The disorder is not attributable to the other varieties of pervasive developmental disorder; acquired aphasia with epilepsy (F80.6); elective mutism (F94.0); Rett's syndrome (F84.2); or schizophrenia (F20.–).

F84.4 Overactive disorder associated with mental retardation and stereotyped movements

A. Severe motor hyperactivity is manifest by at least two of the following problems in activity and attention:

(1) continuous motor restlessness, manifest in running, jumping, and other movements of the whole body;

(2) marked difficulty in remaining seated: the child will ordinarily remain seated for a few seconds at most except when engaged in a stereotypic activity (see criterion B);

(3) grossly excessive activity in situations where relative stillness is expected;

(4) very rapid changes of activity, so that activities generally last for less than a minute (occasional longer periods spent in highly favoured activities do not exclude this, and very long periods spent in stereotypic activities can also be compatible with the presence of this problem at other times).

B. Repetitive and stereotyped patterns of behaviour and activity are manifest by at least one of the following:

(1) fixed and frequently repeated motor mannerisms: these may involve either complex movements of the whole body or partial movements such as hand-flapping;

(2) excessive and non-functional repetition of activities that are constant in form: this may be play with a single object (e.g. running water) or a ritual of activities (either alone or involving other people);

(3) repetitive self-injury.

C. IQ is less than 50.

D. There is no social impairment of the autistic type, i.e. the child must show at least three of the following:
   (1) developmentally appropriate use of eye gaze, expression, and posture to regulate social interaction;
   (2) developmentally appropriate peer relationships that include sharing of interests, activities, etc.;
   (3) approaches to other people, at least sometimes, for comfort and affection;
   (4) ability to share other people's enjoyment at times; other forms of social impairment, e.g. a disinhibited approach to strangers, are compatible with the diagnosis.

E. The disorder does not meet diagnostic criteria for autism (F84.0 and F84.1), childhood disintegrative disorder (F84.3), or hyperkinetic disorders (F90.–).

F84.5 Asperger's syndrome

A. There is no clinically significant general delay in spoken or receptive language or cognitive development. Diagnosis requires that single words should have developed by 2 years of age or earlier and that communicative phrases be used by 3 years of age or earlier. Self-help skills, adaptive behaviour, and curiosity about the environment during the first 3 years should be at a level consistent with normal intellectual development. However, motor milestones may be somewhat delayed and motor clumsiness is usual (although not a necessary diagnostic feature). Isolated special skills, often related to abnormal preoccupations, are common, but are not required for diagnosis.

B. There are qualitative abnormalities in reciprocal social interaction (criteria as for autism).

C. The individual exhibits an unusually intense, circumscribed interest or restricted, repetitive, and stereotyped patterns of behaviour, interests, and activities (criteria as for autism; however it would be less usual for these to include either motor mannerisms or preoccupations with part-objects or non-functional elements of play materials).

D. The disorder is not attributable to the other varieties of pervasive developmental disorder: simple schizophrenia (F20.6); schizotypal disorder (F21); obsessive–compulsive disorder (F42.–); anankastic personality disorder (F60.5); reactive and disinhibited attachment disorders of childhood (F94.1 and F94.2, respectively).

F84.8 Other pervasive developmental disorders

F84.9 Pervasive developmental disorder, unspecified

This is a residual diagnostic category that should be used for disorders which fit the general description for pervasive developmental disorders but in which contradictory findings or a lack of adequate information mean that the criteria for any of the other F84 codes cannot be met.

F88 Other disorders of psychological development

F89 Unspecified disorder of psychological development

F90 – F98
Behavioural and emotional disorders with onset usually occurring in childhood and adolescence

F90 Hyperkinetic disorders

Note: The research diagnosis of hyperkinetic disorder requires the definite presence of abnormal levels of inattention, hyperactivity, and restlessness that are pervasive across situations and persistent over time and that are not caused by other disorders such as autism or affective disorders.

G1. *Inattention.* At least six of the following symptoms of inattention have persisted for at least 6 months, to a degree that is maladaptive and inconsistent with the developmental level of the child:

(1) often fails to give close attention to details, or makes careless errors in schoolwork, work, or other activities;

(2) often fails to sustain attention in tasks or play activities;

(3) often appears not to listen to what is being said to him or her;

(4) often fails to follow through on instructions or to finish schoolwork, chores, or duties in the workplace (not because of oppositional behaviour or failure to understand instructions);

(5) is often impaired in organizing tasks and activities;

(6) often avoids or strongly dislikes tasks, such as homework, that require sustained mental effort;

(7) often loses things necessary for certain tasks or activities, such as school assignments, pencils, books, toys, or tools;

(8) is often easily distracted by external stimuli;

(9) is often forgetful in the course of daily activities.

G2. *Hyperactivity.* At least three of the following symptoms of hyperactivity have persisted for at least 6 months, to a degree that is maladaptive and inconsistent with the developmental level of the child:

(1) often fidgets with hands or feet or squirms on seat;

(2) leaves seat in classroom or in other situations in which remaining seated is expected;

(3) often runs about or climbs excessively in situations in which it is inappropriate (in adolescents or adults, only feelings of restlessness may be present);

(4) is often unduly noisy in playing or has difficulty in engaging quietly in leisure activities;

(5) exhibits a persistent pattern of excessive motor activity that is not substantially modified by social context or demands.

G3. *Impulsivity*. At least one of the following symptoms of impulsivity has persisted for at least 6 months, to a degree that is maladaptive and inconsistent with the developmental level of the child:

(1) often blurts out answers before questions have been completed;

(2) often fails to wait in lines or await turns in games or group situations;

(3) often interrupts or intrudes on others (e.g. butts into others' conversations or games);

(4) often talks excessively without appropriate response to social constraints.

G4. Onset of the disorder is no later than the age of 7 years.

G5. *Pervasiveness*. The criteria should be met for more than a single situation, e.g. the combination of inattention and hyperactivity should be present both at home and at school, or at both school and another setting where children are observed, such as a clinic. (Evidence for cross-situationality will ordinarily require information from more than one source; parental reports about classroom behaviour, for instance, are unlikely to be sufficient.)

G6. The symptoms in G1–G3 cause clinically significant distress or impairment in social, academic, or occupational functioning.

G7. The disorder does not meet the criteria for pervasive developmental disorders (F84.–), manic episode (F30.–), depressive episode (F32.–), or anxiety disorders (F41.–).

Comment

Many authorities also recognize conditions that are sub-threshold for hyperkinetic disorder. Children who meet criteria in other ways but do not show abnormalities of hyperactivity/impulsiveness may be recognized as showing *attention deficit*; conversely, children who fall short of criteria for attention problems but meet criteria in other respects may be recognized as showing *activity disorder*. In the same way, children who meet criteria for only one situation (e.g. only the home or only the classroom) may be regarded as showing a *home-specific* or *classroom-specific disorder*. These conditions are not yet included in the main classification because of insufficient empirical predictive validation, and because many children with sub-threshold disorders show other syndromes (such as oppositional defiant disorder, F91.3) and should be classified in the appropriate category.

F90.0 Disturbance of activity and attention

The general criteria for hyperkinetic disorder (F90) must be met, but not those for conduct disorders (F91.–).

F90.1 Hyperkinetic conduct disorder

The general criteria for both hyperkinetic disorder (F90) and conduct disorders (F91.–) must be met.

F90.8 Other hyperkinetic disorders

F90.9 Hyperkinetic disorder, unspecified

This residual category is not recommended and should be used only when there is a lack of differentiation between F90.0 and F90.1 but the overall criteria for F90.– are fulfilled.

F91 Conduct disorders

G1. There is a repetitive and persistent pattern of behaviour, in which either the basic rights of others or major age-appropriate societal norms or rules are violated, lasting at least 6 months, during which some of the following symptoms are present (see individual subcategories for rules or numbers of symptoms).

Note: The symptoms in 11, 13, 15, 16, 20, 21, and 23 need only have occurred once for the criterion to be fulfilled.

The individual:

(1) has unusually frequent or severe temper tantrums for his or her developmental level;

(2) often argues with adults;

(3) often actively refuses adults' requests or defies rules;

(4) often, apparently deliberately, does things that annoy other people;

(5) often blames others for his or her own mistakes or misbehaviour;

(6) is often "touchy" or easily annoyed by others;

(7) is often angry or resentful;

(8) is often spiteful or vindictive;

(9) often lies or breaks promises to obtain goods or favours or to avoid obligations;

(10) frequently initiates physical fights (this does not include fights with siblings);

(11) has used a weapon that can cause serious physical harm to others (e.g. bat, brick, broken bottle, knife, gun);

(12) often stays out after dark despite parental prohibition (beginning before 13 years of age);

(13) exhibits physical cruelty to other people (e.g. ties up, cuts, or burns a victim);

(14) exhibits physical cruelty to animals;

(15) deliberately destroys the property of others (other than by fire-setting);

(16) deliberately sets fires with a risk or intention of causing serious damage;

(17) steals objects of non-trivial value without confronting the victim, either within the home or outside (e.g. shoplifting, burglary, forgery);

(18) is frequently truant from school, beginning before 13 years of age;

(19) has run away from parental or parental surrogate home at least twice or has run away once for more than a single night (this does not include leaving to avoid physical or sexual abuse);

(20) commits a crime involving confrontation with the victim (including purse-snatching, extortion, mugging);

(21) forces another person into sexual activity;

(22) frequently bullies others (e.g. deliberate infliction of pain or hurt, including persistent intimidation, tormenting, or molestation);

(23) breaks into someone else's house, building, or car.

G2. The disorder does not meet the criteria for dissocial personality disorder (F60.2), schizophrenia (F20.–), manic episode (F30.–), depressive episode (F32.–), pervasive developmental disorders (F84.–), or hyperkinetic disorder (F90.–). (If criteria for emotional disorder (F93.–) are met, the diagnosis should be mixed disorder of conduct and emotions, F92.–.)

It is recommended that the age of onset be specified:

— *childhood onset type*: onset of at least one conduct problem before the age of 10 years;

— *adolescent onset type*: no conduct problems before the age of 10 years.

Specification for possible subdivisions

Authorities differ on the best way of subdividing the conduct disorders, although most agree that the disorders are heterogeneous. For determining prognosis, the severity (indexed by number of symptoms) is a better guide than the precise type of symptomatology. The best-validated distinction is that between *socialized* and *unsocialized* disorders, defined by the presence or absence of lasting peer friendships. However, it seems that disorders confined to the family context may also constitute an important variety, and a category is provided for this purpose. It is clear that further research is needed to test the validity of all proposed subdivisions of conduct disorder.

In addition to these categorizations, it is recommended that cases be described in terms of their scores on three dimensions of disturbance:

(1) hyperactivity (inattentive, restless behaviour);

(2) emotional disturbance (anxiety, depression, obsessionality, hypochondriasis); and

(3) severity of conduct disorder :

(a) *mild*: few if any conduct problems are in excess of those required to make the diagnosis, *and* conduct problems cause only minor harm to others;

(b) *moderate*: the number of conduct problems and the effects on others are intermediate between "mild" and "severe";

(c) *severe*: there are many conduct problems in excess of those required to make the diagnosis, *or* the conduct problems cause considerable harm to others, e.g. severe physical injury, vandalism, or theft.

F91.0 Conduct disorder confined to the family context

A. The general criteria for conduct disorder (F91) must be met.

B. Three or more of the symptoms listed for F91 criterion G1 must be present, with at least three from items (9)–(23).

C. At least one of the symptoms from items (9)–(23) must have been present for at least 6 months.

D. Conduct disturbance must be limited to the family context.

F91.1 Unsocialized conduct disorder

A. The general criteria for conduct disorder (F91) must be met.

B. Three or more of the symptoms listed for F91 criterion G1 must be present, with at least three from items (9)–(23).

C. At least one of the symptoms from items (9)–(23) must have been present for at least 6 months.

D. There must be definitely poor relationships with the individual's peer group, as shown by isolation, rejection, or unpopularity, and by a lack of lasting close reciprocal friendships.

F91.2 Socialized conduct disorder

A. The general criteria for conduct disorder (F91) must be met.

B. Three or more of the symptoms listed for F91 criterion G1 must be present, with at least three from items (9)–(23).

C. At least one of the symptoms from items (9)–(23) must have been present for at least 6 months.

D. Conduct disturbance must include settings outside the home or family context.

E. Peer relationships are within normal limits.

F91.3 Oppositional defiant disorder

A. The general criteria for conduct disorder (F91) must be met.

B. Four or more of the symptoms listed for F91 criterion G1 must be present, but with no more than two symptoms from items (9)–(23).

C. The symptoms in criterion B must be maladaptive and inconsistent with the developmental level.

D. At least four of the symptoms must have been present for at least 6 months.

F91.8 Other conduct disorders

F91.9 Conduct disorder, unspecified

This residual category is not recommended and should be used only for disorders that meet the general criteria for F91 but that have not been specified as to subtype or that do not fulfil the criteria for any of the specified subtypes.

F92 Mixed disorders of conduct and emotions

F92.0 Depressive conduct disorder

A. The general criteria for conduct disorders (F91.–) must be met.

B. Criteria for one of the mood [affective] disorders (F30–39) must be met.

F92.8 Other mixed disorders of conduct and emotions

A. The general criteria for conduct disorders (F91.–) must be met.

B. Criteria for one of the neurotic, stress-related, and somatoform disorders (F40–48) or childhood emotional disorders (F93.–) must be met.

F92.9 Mixed disorder of conduct and emotions, unspecified

F93 Emotional disorders with onset specific to childhood

Note. Phobic anxiety disorder of childhood (F93.1), social anxiety disorder of childhood (F93.2), and general anxiety disorder of childhood (F93.80) have obvious similarities to some of the disorders in F40–F48, but current evidence and opinion suggest that there are sufficient differences in the ways that anxiety disorders present in children for additional categories to be provided. Further studies should show whether descriptions and definitions can be developed that can be used satisfactorily for both adults and children, or whether the present distinction should be preserved.

F93.0 Separation anxiety disorder of childhood

A. At least three of the following must be present:

(1) unrealistic and persistent worry about possible harm befalling major attachment figures or about the loss of such figures (e.g. fear that they will leave and not return or that the child will not see them again), or persistent concerns about the death of attachment figures;

(2) unrealistic and persistent worry that some untoward event will separate the child from a major attachment figure (e.g. the child getting lost, being kidnapped, admitted to hospital, or killed);

(3) persistent reluctance or refusal to go to school because of fear over separation from a major attachment figure or in order to stay at home (rather than for other reasons such as fear over events at school);

(4) difficulty in separating at night, as manifested by any of the following:

(a) persistent reluctance or refusal to go to sleep without being near an attachment figure;

(b) getting up frequently during the night to check on, or to sleep near, an attachment figure;

(c) persistent reluctance or refusal to sleep away from home;

(5) persistent inappropriate fear of being alone, or otherwise without the major attachment figure, at home during the day;

(6) repeated nightmares involving themes of separation;

(7) repeated occurrence of physical symptoms (such as nausea, stomachache, headache, or vomiting) on occasions that involve separation from a major attachment figure, such as leaving home to go to school or on other occasions involving separation (holidays, camps, etc.).

(8) excessive, recurrent distress in anticipation of, during, or immediately following separation from a major attachment figure (as shown by: anxiety, crying, tantrums; persistent reluctance to go away from home; excessive need to talk with parents or desire to return home; misery, apathy, or social withdrawal).

B. The criteria for generalized anxiety disorder of childhood (F93.80) are not met.

C. Onset is before the age of 6 years.

D. The disorder does not occur as part of a broader disturbance of emotions, conduct, or personality, or of a pervasive developmental disorder, psychotic disorder, or psychoactive substance use disorder.

E. Duration of the disorder is at least 4 weeks.

F93.1 Phobic anxiety disorder of childhood

A. The individual manifests a persistent or recurrent fear (phobia) that is developmentally phase-appropriate (or was so at the time of onset) but that is abnormal in degree and is associated with significant social impairment.

B. The criteria for generalized anxiety disorder of childhood (F93.80) are not met.

C. The disorder does not occur as part of a broader disturbance of emotions, conduct, or personality, or of a pervasive developmental disorder, psychotic disorder, or psychoactive substance use disorder.

D. Duration of the disorder is at least 4 weeks.

F93.2 Social anxiety disorder of childhood

A. Persistent anxiety in social situations in which the child is exposed to unfamiliar people, including peers, is manifested by socially avoidant behaviour.

B. The child exhibits self-consciousness, embarrassment, or over-concern about the appropriateness of his or her behaviour when interacting with unfamiliar figures.

C. There is significant interference with social (including peer) relationships, which are consequently restricted; when new or forced social situations are experienced, they cause marked distress and discomfort as manifested by crying, lack of spontaneous speech, or withdrawal from the social situation.

D. The child has satisfying social relationships with familiar figures (family members or peers that he or she knows well).

E. Onset of the disorder generally coincides with a developmental phase where these anxiety reactions are considered appropriate. The abnormal degree, persistence over time, and associated impairment must be manifest before the age of 6 years.

F. The criteria for generalized anxiety disorder of childhood (F93.80) are not met.

G. The disorder does not occur as part of broader disturbances of emotions, conduct, or personality, or of a pervasive developmental disorder, psychotic disorder, or psychoactive substance use disorder.

H. Duration of the disorder is at least 4 weeks.

F93.3 Sibling rivalry disorder

A. The child has abnormally intense negative feelings towards an immediately younger sibling.

B. Emotional disturbance is shown by regression, tantrums, dysphoria, sleep difficulties, oppositional behaviour, or attention-seeking behaviour with one or both parents (two or more of these must be present).

C. Onset is within 6 months of the birth of an immediately younger sibling.

D. Duration of the disorder is at least 4 weeks.

F93.8 Other childhood emotional disorders

F93.80 Generalized anxiety disorder of childhood

Note: In children and adolescents the range of complaints by which the general anxiety is manifest is often more limited than in adults (see F41.1), and the specific symptoms of autonomic arousal are often less prominent. For these individuals, the following alternative set of criteria can be used if preferred:

A. Extensive anxiety and worry (apprehensive expectation) occur on at least half of the total number of days over a period of at least 6 months, the anxiety and worry referring to at least several events or activities (such as work or school performance).

B. The individual finds it difficult to control the worry.

C. The anxiety and worry are associated with at least three of the following symptoms (with at least two symptoms present on at least half of the total number of days):
   (1) restlessness, feeling "keyed up" or "on edge" (as shown, for example, by feelings of mental tension combined with an inability to relax);
   (2) feeling tired, "worn out", or easily fatigued because of worry or anxiety;
   (3) difficulty in concentrating, or mind "going blank";
   (4) irritability;
   (5) muscle tension;
   (6) sleep disturbance (difficulty in falling or staying asleep, or restless, unsatisfying sleep) because of worry or anxiety.

D. The multiple anxieties and worries occur across at least two situations, activities, contexts, or circumstances. Generalized anxiety does not present as discrete paroxysmal episodes (as in panic disorder), nor are the main worries confined to a single, major theme (as in separation anxiety disorder or phobic disorder of childhood). (When more focused anxiety is identified in the broader context of a generalized anxiety, generalized anxiety disorder takes precedence over other anxiety disorders.)

E. Onset occurs in childhood or adolescence (before the age of 18 years).

F. The anxiety, worry, or physical symptoms cause clinically significant distress or impairment in social, occupational, or other important areas of functioning.

G. The disorder is not due to the direct effects of a substance (e.g. psychoactive substances, medication) or a general medical condition (e.g. hyperthyroidism) and does not occur exclusively during a mood disorder, psychotic disorder, or pervasive developmental disorder.

F93.9 Childhood emotional disorder, unspecified

F94 Disorders of social functioning with onset specific to childhood or adolescence

F94.0 Elective mutism

Note. This disorder is also referred to as selective mutism.

A. Language expression and comprehension, as assessed on individually administered standardized tests, is within the 2 standard deviations limit for the child's age.

B. There is demonstrable evidence of a consistent failure to speak in specific social situations in which the child would be expected to speak (e.g. in school), despite speaking in other situations.

C. Duration of the elective mutism exceeds 4 weeks.

D. There is no pervasive developmental disorder (F84.–).

E. The disorder is not accounted for by a lack of knowledge of the spoken language required in the social situation in which there is a failure to speak.

F94.1 Reactive attachment disorder of childhood

A. Onset is before the age of 5 years.

B. The child exhibits strongly contradictory or ambivalent social responses that extend across social situations (but that may show variability from relationship to relationship).

C. Emotional disturbance is shown by lack of emotional responsiveness, withdrawal reactions, aggressive responses to the child's own or other's distress, and/or fearful hypervigilance.

D. Some capacity for social reciprocity and responsiveness is evident in interactions with normal adults.

E. The criteria for pervasive developmental disorders (F84.–) are not met.

F94.2 Disinhibited attachment disorder of childhood

A. Diffuse attachments are a persistent feature during the first 5 years of life (but do not necessarily persist into middle childhood). Diagnosis requires a relative failure to show selective social attachments manifest by:

(1) a normal tendency to seek comfort from others when distressed; and

(2) an abnormal (relative) lack of selectivity in the people from whom comfort is sought.

B. Social interactions with unfamiliar people are poorly modulated.

C. At least one of the following must be present:

(1) generally clinging behaviour in infancy;

(2) attention-seeking and indiscriminately friendly behaviour in early or middle childhood.

D. The general lack of situation-specificity in the above features must be clear. Diagnosis requires that the symptoms in criteria A and B above are manifest across the range of social contacts experienced by the child.

F94.8 Other childhood disorders of social functioning

F94.9 Childhood disorder of social functioning, unspecified

F95 Tic disorders

Note: A tic is an involuntary, sudden, rapid, recurrent, non-rythmic, stereotyped motor movement or vocalization.

F95.0 Transient tic disorder

A. Single or multiple motor or vocal tic(s) or both occur many times a day, on most days, over a period of at least 4 weeks.

B. Duration of the disorder is 12 months or less.

C. There is no history of Tourette syndrome, and the disorder is not the result of physical conditions or side-effects of medication.

D. Onset is before the age of 18 years.

F95.1 Chronic motor or vocal tic disorder

A. Motor or vocal tics, but not both, occur many times per day, on most days, over a period of at least 12 months.

B. No period of remission during that year lasts longer than 2 months.

C. There is no history of Tourette syndrome, and the disorder is not the result of physical conditions or side-effects of medication.

D. Onset is before the age of 18 years.

F95.2 Combined vocal and multiple motor tic disorder [de la Tourette's syndrome]

A. Multiple motor tics and one or more vocal tics have been present at some time during the disorder, but not necessarily concurrently.

B. The frequency of tics must be many times a day, nearly every day, for more that 1 year, with no period of remission during that year lasting longer than 2 months.

C. Onset is before the age of 18 years.

F95.8 Other tic disorders

F95.9 Tic disorder, unspecified

A non-recommended residual category for a disorder that fulfils the general criteria for a tic disorder but in which the specific subcategory is not specified or in which the features do not fulfil the criteria for F95.0, F95.1, or F95.2.

F98 Other emotional and behavioural disorders with onset usually occurring in childhood and adolescence

F98.0 Nonorganic enuresis

A. The child's chronological and mental age is at least 5 years.

B. Involuntary or intentional voiding of urine into bed or clothes occurs at least twice a month in children aged under 7 years, and at least once a month in children aged 7 years or more.

C. The enuresis is not a consequence of epileptic attacks or of neurological incontinence, and not a direct consequence of structural abnormalities of the urinary tract or any other non-psychiatric medical condition.

D. There is no evidence of any other psychiatric disorder that meets the criteria for other ICD-10 categories.

E. Duration of the disorder is at least 3 months.

A fifth character may be used, if desired, for further specification:

F98.00 Nocturnal enuresis only

F98.01 Diurnal enuresis only

F98.02 Nocturnal and diurnal enuresis

F98.1 Nonorganic encopresis

A. The child repeatedly passes faeces in places that are inappropriate for the purpose (e.g. clothing, floor), either involuntarily or intentionally. (The disorder may involve overflow incontinence secondary to functional faecal retention.)

B. The child's chronological and mental age is at least 4 years.

C. There is at least one encopretic event per month.

D. Duration of the disorder is at least 6 months.

E. There is no organic condition that constitutes a sufficient cause for the encopretic events.

A fifth character may be used, if desired, for further specification:

F98.10 Failure to acquire physiological bowel control

F98.11 Adequate bowel control with normal faeces deposited in inappropriate places

F98.12 Soiling associated with excessively fluid faeces (such as with retention with overflow)

F98.2 Feeding disorder of infancy and childhood

A. There is persistent failure to eat adequately, or persistent rumination or regurgitation of food.

B. The child fails to gain weight, loses weight, or exhibits some other significant health problem over a period of at least 1 month. (In view of the frequency of transient eating difficulties, researchers may prefer a minimum duration of 3 months for some purposes.)

C. Onset of the disorder is before the age of 6 years.

D. The child exhibits no other mental or behavioural disorder in the ICD-10 classification (other than mental retardation, F70–F79).

E. There is no evidence of organic disease sufficient to account for the failure to eat.

F98.3 Pica of infancy and childhood

A. There is persistent or recurrent eating of non-nutritive substances, at least twice a week.

B. Duration of the disorder is at least 1 month. (For some purposes, researchers may prefer a minimum period of 3 months.)

C. The child exhibits no other mental or behavioural disorder in the ICD-10 classification (other than mental retardation, F70–F79).

D. The child's chronological and mental age is at least 2 years.

E. The eating behaviour is not part of a culturally sanctioned practice.

F98.4 Stereotyped movement disorders

A. The child exhibits stereotyped movements to an extent that either causes physical injury or markedly interferes with normal activities.

B. Duration of the disorder is at least 1 month.

C. The child exhibits no other mental or behavioural disorder in the ICD-10 classification (other than mental retardation, F70–F79).

A fifth character may be used, if desired, for further specification:

F98.40 Non self-injurious

F98.41 Self-injurious

F98.42 Mixed

F98.5 Stuttering [stammering]

A. Stuttering (i.e. speech characterized by frequent repetition or prolongation of sounds or syllables or words, or by frequent hesitations or pauses) is persistent or recurrent and sufficiently severe to cause marked disruption of the fluency of speech.

B. Duration of the disorder is at least 3 months.

F98.6 Cluttering

A. Cluttering (i.e. rapid speech with breakdown in fluency, but no repetitions or hesitations) is persistent or recurrent and sufficiently severe to reduce significantly the intelligibility of speech.

B. Duration of the disorder is at least 3 months.

F98.8 Other specified behavioural and emotional disorders with onset usually occurring in childhood and adolescence

F98.9 Unspecified behavioural and emotional disorders with onset usually occurring in childhood and adolescence

F99
Unspecified mental disorder

F99 Mental disorder, not otherwise specified

This is a non-recommended residual category, to be employed when no other code from F00–F98 can be used.

ANNEX 1

Provisional criteria for selected disorders

This annex contains criteria for a number of disorders whose clinical or scientific status is still best regarded as uncertain. The disorders have been suggested for inclusion by interested research groups, but it was considered that further research is indicated before they could be regarded as having sufficient international acceptance to merit inclusion in Chapter V(F) of ICD-10. It is hoped that their presence in this annex, with provisional criteria, will stimulate research to clarify their nature and status.

Seasonal affective disorder

(could be applied to mood [affective] disorder, categories F30.–, F31–, F32.– and F33.–)

A. Three or more episodes of mood [affective] disorder must occur, with onset within the same 90-day period of the year, for 3 or more consecutive years.

B. Remissions also occur within a particular 90-day period of the year.

C. Seasonal episodes substantially outnumber any non-seasonal episodes that may occur.

Bipolar II disorder

(could be applied to bipolar affective disorder, categories F31.0, F31.3–F31.5, F31.7)

A. There must be one or more episodes of depression (F32.–).

B. There must be one or more episodes of hypomania (F30.0).

C. There are no episodes of mania (F30.1–F30.2).

Rapid cycling bipolar disorder

(could be applied to bipolar affective disorder, categories F31.0–F31.7)

A. The criteria for bipolar affective disorder, F31.0–F31.7, must be fulfilled.

B. At least four episodes of bipolar affective disorder must occur within a 12-month period

Note: Episodes are demarcated by a switch to an episode of opposite or mixed polarity or by a remission.

Narcissistic personality disorder

A. The general criteria for personality disorder (F60.–) must be fulfilled.

B. The individual must exhibit at least five of the following:

(1) a grandiose sense of self-importance (e.g. the individual exaggerates achievements and talents, expects to be recognized as superior without commensurate achievements);

(2) preoccupation with fantasies of unlimited success, power, brilliance, beauty, or ideal love;

(3) belief that he or she is "special" and unique and can be understood only by, or should associate only with, other special or high-status people (or institutions);

(4) need for excessive admiration;

(5) a sense of entitlement; unreasonable expectations of especially favourable treatment or automatic compliance with his or her expectations;

(6) exploitation of interpersonal relationships, taking advantage of others to achieve his or her own ends;

(7) lack of empathy; unwillingness to recognize or identify with the feelings and needs of others;

(8) frequent envy of others or belief that others are envious of him or her;

(9) arrogant, haughty behaviour or attitudes.

Passive–aggressive (negativistic) personality disorder

A. The general criteria for personality disorder (F60.–) must be met.

B. The individual must exhibit at least five of the following:

(1) procrastination and delay in completing essential, routine tasks, especially those that others seek to have completed;

(2) unjustified protestation that others make unreasonable demands;

(3) sulkiness, irritability, or argumentativeness when the individual is asked to do something he or she does not want to do;

(4) unreasonable criticism of or scorn for people in positions of authority;

(5) deliberately slow or poor work on tasks that the individual really does not want to do;

(6) obstruction of the efforts of others by the individual failing to do his or her share of the work;

(7) avoidance of obligations by claiming to have forgotten.

ANNEX 2

Culture-specific disorders[1]

Culture-specific disorders have diverse characteristics but share two principal features:

(1) they are not easily accommodated by the categories in established and internationally used psychiatric classifications;

(2) they were first described in, and subsequently closely or exclusively associated with, a particular population or cultural area.

These syndromes have also been referred to as culture-bound or culture-reactive, and as ethnic or exotic psychoses. Some are rare and some may be comparatively common; many are acute and transient, which makes their systematic study particularly difficult.

The status of these disorders is controversial: many researchers argue that they differ only in degree from disorders already included in existing psychiatric classifications, such as anxiety disorders and reactions to stress, and that they are therefore best regarded as local variations of disorders that have long been recognized. Their exclusive occurrence in specific population or cultural areas has also been questioned.

There is a clear need for research that will help to establish reliable clinical descriptions of these disorders and clarify their distribution, frequency, and course. In the hope of stimulating and facilitating such research, WHO has undertaken the development of a glossary containing lexical definitions of terms used in cross-cultural and anthropological psychiatric research. It is expected that this glossary will become available in 1994. In the meantime, 12 frequently described "culture-specific" disorders have been included in this annex by way of example, together with their clinical characteristics – extracted from anthropological and medical literature – and suggestions concerning their placement in ICD categories.

No attempt has been made to list detailed diagnostic criteria for these disorders: it is hoped that this will become possible when more reliable clinical, anthropological, epidemiological, and biological information is available.

---

[1] By Dr Ruthbeth Finerman, Associate Professor, Department of Anthropology, Memphis State University, Memphis, TN, USA.

Assignment of the disorders to categories in ICD-10, Chapter V(F), must be regarded as tentative. In certain instances, when available descriptions suggest that there is considerable variation in the clinical states covered by the term, more than one code has been given.

References

Lebra WP, ed. *Culture-bound syndromes, ethnopsychiatry, and alternate therapies.* Honolulu, University of Hawaii, 1976.

Simons RC, Hughes CC, eds. *The culture-bound syndromes.* Dordrecht, Reidel, 1985.

Yap Pow-Meng. Mental diseases peculiar to certain cultures: a survey of comparative psychiatry. *Journal of mental science*, 1951, **97**: 313–327.

Amok (Indonesia; Malaysia)

An indiscriminate, seemingly unprovoked episode of homicidal or highly destructive behaviour, followed by amnesia or fatigue. Many episodes culminate in suicide. Most events occur without warning, although some are precipitated by a period of intense anxiety or hostility. Some studies suggest that cases may derive from the traditional values placed on extreme aggression and suicidal attacks in warfare.

Suggested ICD-10 code

F68.8 Other specified disorders of adult personality and behaviour

Potentially related syndromes

ahade idzi be (the island of New Guinea)
benzi mazurazura (southern Africa (among Shona and affiliated groups))
berserkergang (Scandinavia)
cafard (Polynesia)
colerina (the Andes of Bolivia, Colombia, Ecuador, and Peru)
hwa-byung (Korean peninsula)
iich'aa (indigenous peoples of south-western USA)

References

Lin Keh-Ming. Hwa-byung: a Korean culture-bound syndrome? *American journal of psychiatry*, 1983, **140**(1): 105–107.

Newman P. 'Wild man' behavior in a New Guinea Highlands community. *American anthropologist*, 1964, **66**: 1–19.

Simons RC, Hughes CC, eds. *The culture-bound syndromes*. Dordrecht, Reidel, 1985: 197–264.

Spores J. *Running amok: an historical inquiry*. Athens, OH, Ohio University Center for International Studies, 1988 (Southeast Asia Series, No. 82).

Yap Pow-Meng. The culture-bound reactive syndromes. In: Caudill W, Tsung-yi Lin, eds. *Mental health research in Asia and the Pacific*. Honolulu, East-West Center Press, 1969: 33–53.

Dhat, dhatu, jiryan, shen k'uei, shen-kui (India; China)

Anxiety and somatic complaints such as fatigue and muscle pain, related to a fear of semen loss in men or women (also thought to secrete semen). Precursors are said to include excess coitus, urinary disorders, imbalances in body humours, and diet. The main symptom is a whitish discharge in urine, interpreted as semen loss. Traditional remedies focus on herbal tonics to restore semen or humoral balance.

Suggested ICD-10 codes

F48.8 Other specified neurotic disorders

F45.34 Somatoform autonomic dysfunction of the genitourinary system (may be used if autonomic anxiety symptoms are present)

Potentially related syndromes

koro (China)
rabt (Egypt)

References

Bhatia MS, Malik SC. Dhat syndrome – a useful diagnostic entity in Indian culture. *British journal of psychiatry*, 1991, **159**: 691–695.

Malhotra M, Wig N. Dhat syndrome: a culture-bound sex neurosis of the Orient. *Archives of sexual behavior*, 1975, **4**: 519–528.

Singh SP. Is Dhat culture bound? *British journal of psychiatry*, 1992, **160**: 280–281.

Wen Jung-Kwang, Wang Ching-Lun. Shen-k'uei syndrome: a culture-specific sexual neurosis in Taiwan. In: Kleinman A, Lin Tsung-yi, eds. *Normal and abnormal behavior in Chinese culture*. Dordrecht, Reidel, 1981: 357–369.

Koro, jinjin bemar, suk yeong, suo-yang (south-east Asia, south China, India)

Acute panic or anxiety reaction involving fear of genital retraction. In severe cases, men become convinced that the penis will suddenly withdraw into the abdomen; women sense that their breasts, labia, or vulva will retract. Victims expect the consequences to be fatal. Studies cite factors such as illness, exposure to cold, or excess coitus as precursors, but interpersonal conflict and sociocultural demands reportedly exert greater influence on the condition. Onset is rapid, intense, and unexpected. Responses vary, but include grasping of the genitals by the victim or a family member, application of splints or devices to prevent retraction, herbal remedies, massage, or fellatio.

Suggested ICD-10 codes

F48.8 Other specified neurotic disorders

F45.34 Somatoform autonomic dysfunction of the genitourinary system (may be used if autonomic anxiety symptoms are present)

Potentially related syndromes

dhat (India)

rabt (Egypt)

References

Adityanjee, Zain AM, Subramaniam M. Sporadic koro and marital dysharmony. *Psychopathology*, 1991, **24**(1): 49–52.

Bernstein RL, Gaw AC. Koro: proposed classification for DSM-IV. *American journal of psychiatry*, 1990, **147**(12): 1670–1674.

Nandi DN et al. Epidemic koro in West Bengal, India. *International journal of social psychiatry*, 1983, **29**: 265–268.

Simons RC, Hughes CC, eds. *The culture-bound syndromes*. Dordrecht, Reidel, 1985.

Turnier L, Chouinard G. Effet anti-koro d'un antidépresseur tricyclique. [The anti-koro effect of a tricyclic antidepressant.] *Canadian journal of psychiatry*, 1990, **35**: 331–333.

Latah (Indonesia; Malaysia)

Highly exaggerated responses to a fright or trauma, followed by involuntary echolalia, echopraxia, or trance-like states. Studies variously interpret cases as a neurophysiological response, a hyper-suggestible state, or a mechanism for expressing low self-image. On-lookers usually find such imitative episodes amusing, while victims feel humiliated.

Suggested ICD-10 codes

F48.8 Other specified neurotic disorders
F44.88 Other specified dissociative [conversion] disorders

Potentially related syndromes

amurakh (Siberia)
bah-tsi (Thailand)
imu (Ainu (indigenous people of Japan))
jumping frenchman (Canada)
Lapp panic (Lapps)
mali-mali (Philippines)
pibloktoq (Inuits living within the Arctic Circle)
susto (Mexico, Central and South America)
yaun (Myanmar (formerly Burma))

References

Jenner JA. Latah as coping: a case study offering a new paradox to solve the old one. *International journal of social psychiatry*, 1990, **36**(3): 194–199.

Jenner JA. A successfully treated Dutch case of latah. *Journal of nervous and mental disease*, 1991, **179**(10): 636–637.

Murphy HBM. Notes for a theory on latah. In: Lebra WP, ed. *Culture-bound syndromes, ethnopsychiatry, and alternate therapies*. Honolulu, University of Hawaii, 1976: 3–21.

Simons RC, Hughes CC, eds. *The culture-bound syndromes*. Dordrecht, Reidel, 1985: 41–113.

Nerfiza, nerves, nevra, nervios (Egypt; northern Europe; Greece; Mexico, Central and South America)

Common, often chronic, episodes of extreme sorrow or anxiety, inducing a complex of somatic complaints such as head and muscle pain, diminished reactivity, nausea, appetite loss, insomnia, fatigue, and agitation. The syndrome is more common in women than in men. Research links the condition to stress, anger, emotional distress, and low self-esteem. Cases are traditionally treated with herbal teas, "nerve pills", rest, isolation, and family support.

Suggested ICD-10 codes

F32.11 Moderate depressive episode with somatic syndrome (this is the most likely code)
F48.0 Neurasthenia
F45.1 Undifferentiated somatoform disorder

Potentially related syndromes

anfechtung (Hutterites (a religious group))
brain fag (Nigeria)
colerina, pension, bilis (Mexico, Central and South America)
hsieh-ping, xie-bing (China)
hwa-byung (Korean peninsula)
narahati-e a sab, maraz-e a sab (Islamic Republic of Iran)
qissaatuq (Inuits living within the Arctic Circle)

References

Historical and cross-cultural perspectives on nerves. *Social science and medicine*, 1988, **26**(12): 1197–1259.

Davis DL, Low SM, eds. *Gender, health and illness: the case of nerves*. New York, Hemisphere, 1989.

Good B, Good MJD, Moradi R. The interpretation of Iranian depressive illness and dysphoric affect. In: Kleinman A, Good B, eds. *Culture and depression*. Berkeley, University of California, 1985: 369–428.

Low SM. Culturally interpreted symptoms or culture-bound syndromes: a cross-cultural review of nerves. *Social science and medicine*, 1985, **21**(2): 187–196.

Pa-leng, frigophobia (China (Province of Taiwan); south-east Asia)

Anxiety state characterized by obsessive fear of cold and winds, believed to produce fatigue, impotence, or death. Victims compulsively dress in heavy or excessive clothing. Fears are reinforced by cultural views of the condition as a legitimate humoral disorder.

Suggested ICD-10 code

F40.2 Specific phobias

Potentially related syndromes

agua frio, aire frio, frio (Mexico, Central and South America)

References

Kiev A. *Transcultural psychiatry*. New York, Free Press, 1972.

Lin Keh-Ming, Kleinman A, Lin Tsung-Yi. Overview of mental disorders in Chinese cultures: review of epidemiological and clinical studies. In: Kleinman A, Lin Tsung-Yi, eds. *Normal and abnormal behavior in Chinese culture*. Dordrecht, Reidel, 1981: 237–272.

Pibloktoq, Arctic hysteria (Inuits living within the Arctic Circle)

Prodromal fatigue, depression, or confusion, followed by a "seizure" of disruptive behaviour, including stripping or tearing off clothes, frenzied running, rolling in snow, glossolalia or echolalia, echopraxia, property destruction, and coprophagia. Most episodes last only minutes and are followed by loss of consciousness, amnesia, and complete remission. Injury is rare and, while some studies have related cause to hypocalcaemic tetany, most researchers link incidents to interpersonal anxieties and cultural stressors.

Suggested ICD-10 codes

F44.7 Mixed dissociative [conversion] disorders
F44.88 Other specified dissociative [conversion] disorders

Potentially related syndromes

amok (Indonesia; Malaysia)
banga, misala (Congo; Malawi (formerly Nyasaland)
ebenzi (southern Africa, among Shona and affiliated groups)
grisi siknis (Miskito (indigenous people of Honduras))
imu (Ainu (indigenous people of Japan))
latah (Indonesia; Malaysia)
mali-mali (Philippines)
nangiarpok, kayak angst, quajimaillituq (Inuits)
ufufuyane (southern Africa, especially among Bantu, Zulu, and affiliated groups)

References

Parker S. Eskimo psychopathology in the context of Eskimo personality and culture. *American anthropologist*, 1962, **64**: 76–96.

Simons RC, Hughes CC, eds. *The culture-bound syndromes*. Dordrecht, Reidel, 1985: 267–326.

Wallace A. Mental illness, biology and culture. In: Hsu FLK, ed. *Psychological anthropology*. Cambridge, MA, Schenkman, 1972: 363–402.

Susto, espanto (Mexico, Central and South America)

Highly diverse, chronic complaints attributed to "soul loss" induced by a severe, often supernatural, fright. In some cases, traumatic events are not personally experienced; individuals may be stricken when others (usually relatives) suffer a fright. Symptoms often include agitation, anorexia, insomnia, fever, diarrhoea, mental confusion and apathy, depression, and introversion. Studies variously attribute cases to hypoglycaemia, nonspecific organic disease, generalized anxiety, and stress resulting from social conflict and low self-esteem.

Suggested ICD-10 codes

F45.1 Undifferentiated somatoform disorder
F48.8 Other specified neurotic disorders

Potentially related syndromes

lanti (Philippines)
latah (Indonesia; Malaysia)
malgri (aborigines of Australia)
mogo laya (the island of New Guinea)
narahati (Islamic Republic of Iran)
saladera (regions around Amazon river)

References

Good B, Good MJD. Toward a meaning-centered analysis of popular illness categories: fright illness and heart distress in Iran. In: Marsella AJ, White GM, eds. *Cultural conceptions of mental health and therapy*. Dordrecht, Reidel, 1982: 150–158.

Houghton A, Boersma F. The grief-loss connection in susto. *Ethnology*, 1988, **27**: 145–154.

Lipp F. The study of disease in relation to culture — the susto complex among the Mixe of Oaxaca. *Dialectical anthropology*, 1989, **12**: 435–443.

Rubel AJ, O'Nell CW, Collado-Ardon R. *Susto, a folk illness*. Berkeley, University of California Press, 1984.

Simons RC, Hughes CC, eds. *The culture-bound syndromes*. Dordrecht, Reidel, 1985: 329–407.

Taijin kyofusho, shinkeishitsu, anthropophobia (Japan)

Anxiety or phobia more common among men and young adults. Cases are marked by a fear of social contact (especially friends), extreme self-consciousness (concern about physical appearance, body odour, blushing), and a fear of contracting disease. Somatic symptoms include head, body, and stomach aches, fatigue, and insomnia. Victims, popularly regarded as highly intelligent and creative, may display perfectionist tendencies. Studies suggest cultural values encourage "over-socialization" of some children, producing feelings of inferiority and anxiety in social situations.

Suggested ICD-10 codes

F40.1 Social phobias
F40.8 Other phobic anxiety disorders
(may be used if there are many other fears)

Potentially related syndromes

anfechtung (Hutterites (a religious group))
itiju (Nigeria)

References

Lock M. *East Asian medicine in urban Japan*. Berkeley, University of California Press, 1980: 222–224.

Tanaka-Matsumi J. Taijin kyofusho. *Culture, medicine and psychiatry*, 1979, **3**: 231–245.

Prince R, Techeng-Laroche F. Culture bound syndromes and international classification of disease. *Culture, medicine and psychiatry*, 1987, **11**: 3–20.

Reynolds D. *Morita therapy*. Berkeley, University of California Press, 1976.

Ufufuyane, saka (southern Africa (among Bantu, Zulu, and affiliated groups); Kenya)

An anxiety state popularly attributed to magical potions administered by rejected lovers, or spirit possession. Features include shouting, sobbing, repeated neologisms, paralysis, convulsions, and a trance-like stupor or loss of consciousness. Most victims are young, unmarried women. Some experience nightmares with sexual themes or rare episodes of temporary blindness. Attacks, which can continue for days or weeks, may be provoked by the sight of men or foreigners.

Suggested ICD-10 codes

F44.3 Trance and possession disorders
F44.7 Mixed dissociative [conversion] disorders

Potentially related syndromes

aluro (Nigeria)
phii pob (Thailand)
zar (Egypt; Ethiopia; Sudan)

References

Harris G. Possession 'hysteria' in a Kenya tribe. *American anthropologist*, 1957, **59**: 1046–1066.

Loudon JB. Psychogenic disorder and social conflict among the Zulu. In: Opler MK, ed. *Culture and mental health.* New York, Macmillan, 1959: 351–369.

Uqamairineq (Inuits living within the Arctic Circle)

Sudden paralysis associated with borderline sleep states, accompanied by anxiety, agitation, or hallucinations. Prodromal indicators may include a detectable yet transient sound or smell. While the condition is usually chronic and can prompt panic, most attacks last only minutes and are followed by complete remission. Cases are fairly common, and traditionally alleged to result from soul loss, soul wandering, or spirit possession. Studies describe the experience as a dissociative hysterical reaction and possible variant of the narcolepsy–cataplexy syndrome.

Suggested ICD-10 codes

F44.88 Other specified dissociative [conversion] disorders
G47.4 Narcolepsy and cataplexy
Includes: sleep paralysis

Potentially related syndromes

aluro (Nigeria)
old hag (Newfoundland)
phii pob (Thailand)

References

Hufford D. *The terror that comes in the night*. Philadelphia, University of Pennsylvania, 1982.

Parker S. Eskimo psychopathology in the context of Eskimo personality and culture. *American anthropologist*, 1962, **64**: 76–96.

Simons RC, Hughes CC, eds. *The culture-bound syndromes*. Dordrecht, Reidel, 1985: 115–148.

Windigo (various spellings) (indigenous people of north-eastern regions of North America)

Rare, historic accounts of cannibalistic obsession. Traditionally, cases were ascribed to possession, with victims (usually male) turning into cannibal monsters. Symptoms included depression, homicidal or suicidal thoughts, and a delusional, compulsive wish to eat human flesh. Most victims were socially ostracized or put to death. Early research described episodes as hysterical psychosis, precipitated by chronic food shortages and cultural myths about starvation and windigo monsters. Some controversial new studies question the syndrome's legitimacy, claiming cases were actually a product of hostile accusations invented to justify the victim's ostracism or execution.

Suggested ICD-10 code

The available information is too unreliable to suggest a likely code. If a code is needed, use:

F68.8 Other specified disorders of adult personality and behaviour

Potentially related syndromes

amok (Malaysia)
hsieh-ping (China (Province of Taiwan))
zar (Egypt; Ethiopia; Sudan)

References

Bishop C. Northern Algonkian cannibalism and windigo psychosis. In: Williams T, ed. *Psychological anthropology*, The Hague, Mouton, 1975: 237–248.

Hay T. The windigo psychosis. *American anthropologist*, 1971, **73**: 1–19.

Parker S. The wiitiko psychosis in the context of Ojibwa personality and culture. *American anthropologist*, 1960, **62**: 603–623.

Simons RC, Hughes CC, eds. *The culture-bound syndromes*. Dordrecht, Reidel, 1985: 409–465.

List of individual experts

The following list contains the names of experts who were involved in the drafting of this text or whose comments were most useful in refining the research criteria.

Dr G. Andrews, Darlinghurst, Australia
Dr J. Angst, Zurich, Switzerland
Dr T. Babor, Farmington, CT, USA
Dr J. Bancroft, Edinburgh, Scotland
Dr F. Benson, Los Angeles, CA, USA
Dr F. Bianco, Caracas, Venezuela
Dr J. Burke, Temple, TX, USA
Dr D. Cantwell, Los Angeles, CA, USA
Dr S.M. Channabasavanna, Bangalore, India
Dr H. Christensen, Canberra, Australia
Dr A. Clare, London, England
Dr W. Compton, St Louis, MO, USA
Dr J.E. Cooper, Nottingham, England
Dr J.A. Corbett, London, England
Dr L. Cottler, St Louis, MO, USA
Dr W. Eicher, Mannheim, Germany
Dr J. Escobar, Farmington, CT, USA
Dr W. Feuerlein, Munich, Germany
Dr R. García, Santo Domingo, Dominican Republic
Dr M.G. Gelder, Oxford, England
Dr R. Giel, Groningen, Netherlands
Dr J. Glatzel, Mainz, Germany
Dr A. Göğüş, Ankara, Turkey
Dr D. Goldberg, Manchester, England
Dr M. Gossop, London, England
Dr P. Graham, London, England
Dr J. Griffith Edwards, London, England
Dr L. Gustafson, Lund, Sweden
Dr S. Guze, St Louis, MO, USA
Dr H. Häfner, Mannheim, Germany
Dr B. Hagberg, Gothenburg, Sweden
Dr J. Helzer, St Louis, MO, USA
Dr A.S. Henderson, Canberra, Australia
Dr R.M.A. Hirschfeld, Galveston, TX, USA
Dr P. Holzman, Cambridge, MA, USA
Dr Y. Honda, Tokyo, Japan
Dr M. Isaac, Bangalore, India
Dr A. Janca, Geneva, Switzerland
Dr R. Jegede, Ibadan, Nigeria
Dr A.F. Jorm, Canberra, Australia
Dr E.G. Karam, Beirut, Lebanon
Dr R.E. Kendell, Edinburgh, Scotland
Dr A. Kleinman, Cambridge, MA, USA
Dr G.-E. Kühne, Jena, Germany
Dr D. J. Kupfer, Pittsburgh, PA, USA

Dr W.A. Lishman, London, England
Dr Z. Lipowski, Toronto, Canada
Dr J. Lokar, Ljubljana, Slovenia
Dr. A.W. Loranger, White Plains, NY, USA
Dr U. Malt, Oslo, Norway
Dr M. Maj, Naples, Italy
Dr I. Marks, London, England
Dr V. Mavreas, Athens, Greece
Dr J. Mezzich, Pittsburgh, PA, USA
Dr R. Misès, Paris, France
Dr R.A. Nadzharov, Moscow, Russian Federation
Dr J.S. Neki, Dar es Salaam, United Republic of Tanzania
Dr R. Onyango Sumba, Nairobi, Kenya
Dr J. Orley, Geneva, Switzerland
Dr E.S. Paykel, Cambridge, England
Dr C. Perris, Umea, Sweden
Dr L. Robins, St Louis, MO, USA
Dr M. Rubio-Stipec, San Juan, Puerto Rico
Dr G. Russel, London, England
Dr M. Rutter, London, England
Dr B.I. Sacks, London, England
Dr J.B. Saunders, Sydney, Australia
Dr C. Scharfetter, Zurich, Switzerland
Dr P. Sindelar, Geneva, Switzerland
Dr M.A. Schuckit, San Diego, CA, USA
Dr Shen Yu-cun, Beijing, China
Dr M. Shepherd, London, England
Dr Shu Liang, Beijing, China
Dr R. Smeets, Amsterdam, Netherlands
Dr A.B. Smulevitch, Moscow, Russian Federation
Dr C.R. Soldatos, Athens, Greece
Dr R. Spitzer, New York, NY, USA
Dr E. Strömgren, Aarhus, Denmark *(deceased)*
Dr H. Strotzka, Vienna, Austria
Dr E. Taylor, London, England
Dr M. Thorpy, Dunedin, New Zealand
Dr C. Torres de Mirando, São Paulo, Brazil
Dr G.J. Tucker, Seattle, WA, USA
Dr T.B. Üstün, Geneva, Switzerland
Dr J.L. Vazquez-Barquero, Santander, Spain
Dr J.K. Walsh, Rochester, MN, USA
Lord Walton of Detchant, Oxford, England
Dr D.J. West, Cambridge, England
Dr J. Wing, London, England
Dr L. Wing, London, England
Dr H.-U. Wittchen, Munich, Germany
Dr Xu You-xin, Beijing, China

List of field trial coordinating centres, field trial centres reporting to them, and investigators

The names of the field trial coordinating centres are arranged in alphabetical order of their locations (Bangalore, Cairo, etc.).

The field trial centres reporting to a particular coordinating centre are arranged in alphabetical order of the country and then the city of their location.

The names of the directors of field trial centres are marked with an asterisk.

Field trial centres reporting to Bangalore, India

Coordinating centre

National Institute of Mental Health and Neurosciences, Bangalore
Dr C.R. Chandrashekar
*Dr S. Channabasavanna
Dr S. Chatterji
Dr S. Girimaji
Mr M.K. Isaac
Dr S. Jain
Dr S. Khanna
Dr K. Kumar
Dr R. Mehta
Dr R.S. Murthy
Dr R. Raghuram
Dr S. Rao
Dr C. Shamsundar
Dr S. Sheshadri
Dr R. Srinath
Dr T.G. Sriram
Dr M. Verghese

Reporting centres

All-India Institute of Medical Sciences, New Delhi, India
Dr K. Chandirami
Dr S. Dube
Dr V. Kapur
Dr R. Lal
Dr D. Mohan
*Dr S. Saxena

Burnpur Hospital, West Bengal, India
*Dr B. Sen

Christian Medical College, Vellore, India
*Dr J. John
Dr T.M. Kumar

King George's Medical College, Lucknow, India
*Dr A.K. Agarwal
Dr M. Katiyar

Dr S. Kumar
Dr P. Silhatey
Dr H. Singh
Dr J.K. Trivedi

RNT Medical College, Udaipur, India
*Dr L.N. Gupta
Dr D.M. Mathur

Field trial centres reporting to Cairo, Egypt

Coordinating centre

Institute of Psychiatry, Ain Shams University, Cairo
Dr S. Effat
Dr M.R. El Fiki
Dr M. Ghanem
Dr A.H. Khalil
Dr N. Mahawalli
*Dr A. Okasha
Dr M. Refaat
Dr A. Seif El Dawla
Dr A. Shohdi

Reporting centres

Bahrain
Psychiatric Hospital, Manama
*Dr M.K. Al Haddad
Dr C. Kamel
Dr M.A. Karim
Dr M. Kashaba
Dr A. Nabi
Dr O. Saleh
Dr A. Shooka

Egypt
East Town Hospital, Alexandria
Dr N. Fouda
Dr M. Mickael
*Dr S. Nicolas

Maamoura Psychiatric Hospital, Alexandria
Dr E.K. Ahmed
*Dr K. El Fawal
Dr M.F. Wagdi

Lebanon
St George's Hospital, Beirut
*Dr E.G. Karam
Dr P.F. Yabroudi

Morocco
Centre Psychiatrique, Universitaire Ibn Roshd, Casablanca
Dr N. Kadri
*Dr D. Moussaoui
Dr M. Touhaii

Tunisia
Centre Hôpital-Universitaire, Monastir
Dr B. Hatem
*Dr T. Skihiri

United Arab Emirates
U.A.E. University, Al Ain
*Dr T.K. Daradhek
Dr A. Saad

Rashid Hospital, Dubai
Dr A.S. El Din
*Dr E.H. Ghoz

Field trial centres reporting to Lübeck, Germany

Coordinating centre

Klinik für Psychiatrie der Medizinischen Hochschule, Lübeck, Germany
Dr G. Arentewicz
Dr V. Arolt
Dr A. Beknisch
Dr H.-G. Brinkmann
*Dr H. Dilling

Dr M. Driessen
*Dr H.J. Freyberger
Dr U. John
Dr R.-D. Kanitz
Dr S. Kleinschmidt
Dr U. Krippendorf
Dr T. Lefèbre
Dr R. Michels
Dr T. Müller-Thomsen
Dr H. Neubauer
Dr S. Nowak
Dr U. Schüffelgen
Dr E. Schulte-Markwort
Dr A. Schürmann
Dr W. Seibert
Dr U. Siebel
Dr D. Steege
Dr C. Veltrup
Dr T. Wetterling

Reporting centres

Austria

Universitätsklinik für Neuropsychiatrie des Kindes- und Jugendalters, Vienna
*Dr F. Resch

Germany

Psychiatrische Klinik des Rheinisch-Westfälische technische Hochschule Aachen, Aachen
Dr H. Ebel
Dr S. Herpertz
Dr C. Menges
Dr A. Pirad
*Dr H. Sass
Dr H. Zimmer
Dr J. Zimmermann

Abteilung für Gerontopsychiatrie der Psychiatrischen Klinik und Poliklinik der Freien Universität, Berlin
*Dr H. Gutzmann
Dr H. Krüger

Psychiatrische Klinik und Poliklinik der Freien Universität Berlin, Berlin
Dr A. Aggias
Dr M. Bauer
Dr F. Bögner
Dr D. Bolk-Weischedel
Dr C. Brockhaus
Dr Carstens
Dr T.R. Drochner
Dr J.S. Englert
Dr S. Englert
Dr Frota
Dr W. Gaebel
Dr R. Gebhardt
Dr Geiselmann
Dr Gruneberg
Dr R. Hellweg
*Dr H. Helmchen
Dr Hosten
Dr M. Lemke
Dr M. Linden
Dr Loos
Dr A. Mackert
Dr C. Nehrig
Dr M. Otto
Dr A. Pietzcker
Dr J. Podschos
Dr U. Polzer
Dr F. Reischeis
Dr A. Rolfs
Dr T. Sander
Dr L. Schmidt
Dr B. Stotzek
Dr T. Steckler
Dr R.-D. Stieglitz
Dr M. Stöver
Dr G. Streb
Dr K. Thies
Dr M. Ufert
Dr T. Wernicke
Dr C. Wildgrube
Dr T. Wünscher

Klinik für Psychosomatik und Psychotherapie der Westfälischen Klinik für Psychiatrie in Dortmund, Dortmund
Dr H. Bast
Dr M. Becker
Dr P. Bösser
*Dr P. Janssen
Dr K. Martin
Dr H. Rath
Dr K. Rodewig
Dr W. Schneider
Dr M. Tetzlaff
Dr W. Wach

Allgemeine Psychiatrie der Landes- und Hochschulklinik, Essen
*Dr M. Gastpar
Dr C. Rösinger

Klinik für Psychotherapie und Psychosomatik der Rheinischen Landes- und Hochschulklinik, Essen
Dr G. Heuft
*Dr J. van Wyk

Abteilung für Kinder- und Jugendpsychiatrie am Zentrum Psychiatrie der Johann-Wolfgang-Goethe-Universität, Frankfurt-am-Main
Dr S. Denner
Dr E. Englert
Dr K. Koepsell
Dr B. Meyenburg
*Dr F. Poustka
Dr D. Rühl
Dr S. Schlüter-Müller
Dr K. Schmecl
Dr G. Schmötzer

Gelderlandklinik - Fachklinik für Psychotherapie und Psychosomatik, Geldern
*Dr R. Kriebel

Klinik für Psychosomatik und Psychotherapie der Justus-Liebig-Universität, Giessen
*Dr B. Brosig
Dr R. Woidera

Abteilung für Psychosomatik und Psychotherapie der Universität Göttingen, Göttingen
Dr C. Breuer
Dr A. Eckhof
Dr J. Konemann
Dr E. Leibing
*Dr U. Rüger
Dr H. Schauenburg
Dr G. Schlüssler
Dr M. Wächter
Dr A. Weddige-Diederichs

Psychiatrische Klinik der Universität Göttingen, Göttingen
Dr J. Grefe
*Dr E. Rüther
Dr A. Thiel

Abteilung für Psychosomatik der Medizinischen Hochschule Hannover, Hannover
Dr B. Albert
Dr U. Gast
Dr A. Kersting
Dr H.-W. Künsebeck
Dr W. Lempa
*Dr R. Liedtke
Dr I. Reimer
Dr G. Schmidt

Psychosomatische Klinik der Ruprechts-Universität, Heidelberg
*Dr G. Heuft
Dr A. Öri

Klinik für Psychiatrie und Neurologie "Hans Berger", Jena (in cooperation with the psychiatric departments in Hildburghausen and Mühlhausen)
Dr Aber
Dr Auert
Dr Barnstorf
Dr Bauer
Dr Bertram
Dr Dietrich
Dr Dörz
Dr Fehlow
Dr Fischer

Dr Franke
Dr Fritzsche
Dr Fröhlich
Dr F. Häger
Dr Heins
Dr Hoffmann
Dr Johns
Dr H. Kozian
Dr Krause
Dr G.-E. Kühne
Dr Lagmann
Dr Langbein
Dr Lemke
Dr Lesser
Dr Lobenstein
Dr Misselwitz
Dr Otto
Dr Peter
Dr Reitler
Dr Roselt
Dr Schmidt
Dr Schuber
Dr Schwertfeger
Dr Seelisch
Dr Siegel
Dr Tawana
Dr Tschiersch
Dr Warnke
Dr Wünscher

Klinik für Kinder- und Jugendpsychiatrie der Medizinischen Universität, Lübeck
Dr H. Cyganek-Hartwig
Dr A. Harmani-Ochynski
Dr R. Hoppenkamps
*Dr U. Knölker
Dr M. Lücke
Dr M. Neuhauss
Dr G. Roosen-Runge
Dr W. Ruhlender
Dr A. Schneider
Dr M. Schulte-Markwort

Dr E. Sochaczewsky
Dr T. Zenkl

Klinik für Psychosomatik der Medizinischen Universität Lübeck, Lübeck
Dr H. Federschmidt
Dr H. Feiereis
*Dr G. Jantschek
Dr I. Jantschek
Dr H.-G. Kollra
Dr K. Langner
Dr S. Marks-Mitusch
Dr B. Mensing
Dr M. Pollak
Dr B. Probst
Dr J. Redmann
Dr B. Scheferling
Dr R. Schichtling
Dr M. Sudeck
Dr I. Trotno
Dr J. von Wietersheim
Dr E. Wilke
Dr R. Zehendner

Klinik für Psychosomatische Medizin und Psychoanalyse am Zentralinstitut für Seelische Gesundheit, Mannheim
Dr M. Frans
Dr H. Käfer
Dr H.-D. Kortendieck
Dr A. Kriebel
Dr K. Lieberz
Dr M. Markstein
*Dr A. Muhs
*Dr H. Schepank
Dr M. Schierer
Dr A. Schiller
Dr Weber

Klinik für Kinder- and Jugendpsychiatrie der Universität Marburg, Marburg
*Dr B. Herpertz-Dahlmann
Dr K. Quaschner
Dr E. Schulz

Poliklinik der Max-Planck-Instituts für Psychiatrie, Munich
Dr J. Guldner
Dr F. Helgenberger
*Dr W. Mombour
Dr M. Oechsner
Dr T. Pätzold
Dr T. Schier
Dr F.-E. Seier
Dr H. Unland
Dr T. Wetter

Psychiatrisches Abteilung, Krankenhaus Haar, Haar bei München, Munich
*Dr M. Albus
Dr J. Baruth-Krischel
Dr E. Dietzfelbinger
Dr C. Hummel
Dr P. Lauer
Dr G. Scheibe
Dr E. Stiasny

Psychiatrische Klinik und Poliklinik der Ludwig-Maximilians-Universität, Munich
*Dr P. Hoff

Abteilung für Kinderneuropsychiatrie der Universitätsnervenklinik Rostock, Rostock
*Dr H. Camman

Psychiatrische Klinik der Universität, Rostock
Dr B. Dreves
*Dr K. Ernst
Dr K. Friemert
Dr C. Lehmann
Dr R. Mau
Dr C. Rehn
Dr D. Roether
Dr D. Schläfke

Psychotherapeutische Klinik, Krankenhaus für Analytische Psychotherapie und Psychosomatik, Stuttgart
Dr K.-U. Adam
Dr J. Dittert
Dr W. Ehlers
Dr G. Eichner

Dr R. Hettinger
Dr I. Rothe-Kirchberger
Dr T. Seifert
*Dr G. Schmitt
Dr J.-M. Voigtländer

Klinik Berus - Zentrum für Psychosomatik und Verhaltensmedizin, Überherrn-Berus
Dr W. Bürger
Dr A. Dinger-Broda
Dr W. Engelhardt
Dr A. Herrmann
*Dr W. Köhl
Dr W. Miller
Dr P. Osterziel
Dr S. Rittmann
Dr J. Schwickerath
Dr J. Seifert-Haves
Dr T. Stau
Dr C. Thissen
Dr S. Tonscheidt
Dr R. Winter
Dr P. Zenner

Switzerland
Psychiatrische Klinik der Universität Basel, Basel
*Dr V. Dittmann

Poliklinik für Kinder und Jugendliche, Zurich
*Dr H.C. Steinhausen

Field trial centres reporting to Luxembourg

Coordinating centre

Service de Neuro-psychiatrie, Centre Hospitalier de Luxembourg, Luxembourg
Dr C. Ghaillet
*Dr C. Pull

Reporting centres

Belgium

Hôpital Erasme, Brussels
Dr P. Hubain
Dr I. Ramallo Pallast
*Dr L. Staner

France

Clinique Psychiatrique Jérome Bosch, Armentières
Dr V. Garcin
Dr C. Gignac
Dr M. Gomes
Dr A. Gurdal
Dr D. Ochin
Dr B. Parmentier
*Dr J.-L. Roelandt
Dr C. Vosgien

Centre Hospitalier de Cayenne, Cayenne
*Dr E. Aronica
Dr G. Simart

Centre Hospitalier Spécialisé Le Vinatier, Lyon
Dr T. Faivre
Dr N. Georgieff
Dr J.M. Guillaud-Bataille
*Dr M. Marie-Cardine
Dr G. Mecheri
*Dr J.L. Terra

Centre Hospitalier Spécialisé La Verrière, Le Mesnil-St-Denis
*Dr V. Kovess

Centre Hospitalier Specialisé de Colson, Fort-de-France, Martinique
Dr A. Bottius
Dr X. Bouveresse
Dr P. Guillard
Dr G. Gruel
*Dr G. Ursulet

Clinique de Psychiatrie, Nice
Dr B. Bensmail
Dr T. Braccini
*Dr G. Darcourt

Cliniques des Maladies Mentales, Paris
Dr V. Gaillac
*Dr J.D. Guelfi
Dr M.L. Seror

Hôpital Necker, Paris
Dr X. Abillon
*Dr B. Granger

Hôpital Robert Debré, Paris
Dr A.M. Badoual
Dr M. Bouvard
*Dr M. Dugas
Dr X. George
Dr C. Gerard
Dr M. Legendreux
Dr M.F. Le Heuzey

Hôpital de la Salpêtrière, Paris
Dr U. Barua
*Dr A. Lazartigues
Dr H. Morales

Centre Hospitalier Spécialisé du Rouvray, Rouen
Dr F. Besse
Dr P. Brazo
*Dr S. Dollfus
Dr P. Preterre

Hôpital de Bellevue, Saint-Etienne
Dr C. Digonnet
Dr D.G. Froissart
Dr A. Guillot
Dr F. Lang
Dr F. Manipoud
Dr M. Marcon
*Dr J. Pellet

Dr M. Pichon
Dr M.G. Pichon
Dr C. Rascle
Dr X. Tatu

Centre Médico-Psychologique, Saint-Germain-en-Laye
Dr U. Barua
*Dr A.-P. Van Amerongen
Dr S. Virecoulon

Centre Hospitalier Universitaire, Strasbourg
Dr S. Peretti
*Dr L. Singer
Dr M.A. Zimmermann

Israel
Hôpital Psychiatrique Geha, Tel Aviv
Dr M. Danon
Dr M. Granek
Dr M. Radwan
*Dr S. Tyano

Switzerland
Clinique de Psychiatrie, Geneva
Dr E. Bishara
Dr P. Huguelet
*Dr I. Zabala

Clinique Psychiatrique, Lausanne
Dr D. Baettig
Dr J. Besson
Dr C. Bryois
*Dr F. Ferrero
Dr C. Schnyder

Field trial centres reporting to Madrid, Spain

Coordinating centre

Clinica López-Ibor, Madrid
Dr M. Crespo
Dr F. Ferre

*Dr J.J. López-Ibor Jr
Dr L.I. Jordá
Dr J. Saíz Ruiz
Dr M. Vega

Reporting centres

Chile

Clínica Psiquiátrica Universitaria, Universidad de Chile, Santiago
Dr R. Chaparro
Dr B. Díaz Vargas
*Dr F. Lolas
Mrs A. Montenegro
Dr L. Risco
Dr C. Tchimino
Dr C. Téllez
Mrs E. Varela
Mr S. Véliz

Spain

Servicio di Psiquiatría, Hospital del Valle de Hebrón, Barcelona
Dr E. Miró
Dr L.A. Morales
Dr E. Rojo
Dr P. Salgado
Dr J.A. Sanz
Dr J. Serrallonga
*Dr J. Vallejo

Psychiatric Unit, Hospital de la Santa Creu y Sant Pau, Barcelona
*Dr J.C. Pérez de los Cobos
Dr C. Pinet
Dr M.L. Soto

Servicio de Psiquiatría, Ciudad Sanitaria La Paz, Madrid
Dr M.C. Bayón
Dr J. Bellot
Dr F. Cañas
Dr M.C. Culebro Fernández
Dr C. de Dios

Dr B. Franco
Dr R. García Pérez
Dr G. Gómez Mújica
Dr F.R. González-Nicolás
Dr M. Graell
Dr J.J. Martínez García
Dr F. Orengo
Dr B. Rodríguez Vega
*Dr J. Santo Domingo
Dr M.L. Soto

Servicio de Salud Mental, Comunidad de Madrid, Madrid
Dr A. Castaño Romero
*Dr V. Corces Pando
Dr C. González
Dr R. Gutierrez Labrador
Dr M.L. López Girones
Dr C. Polo Usaola
Dr A. Roig Moliner
Dr A. Tejeda Rivas
Dr B. Viar Lahera

Servicio de Salud Mental, Principado de Asturias, Oviedo
*Dr V. Aparicio
Dr B. Cid
Dr G. García
Mrs S. García Tardón
Dr A. González
Dr F. González Aria
Dr S. Ocio Léon
Dr C. Pedrero
Dr E. Peñuela
Dr A. Rincón

Servicio de Psiquiatría, Universidad de Oviedo, Oviedo
*Dr J. Bobes García
Dr P. Gonzáles G. Portilla

Field trial centres reporting to Moscow, Russian Federation

Coordinating centre

Institute of Psychiatry, Academy of Medical Sciences, Moscow
Dr K. Kostyukova
*Dr S. Tzirkin
Dr O. Valova

Field trial centres reporting to Nagasaki, Japan

Coordinating centre

Nagasaki University, Nagasaki
Dr J. Kubota
*Dr Y. Nakane
Dr Y. Okazaki
Dr K. Takada

Reporting centres

Fukui Medical School, Fukui
Dr T. Hayashi
*Dr K. Isaki
Dr Y. Koshino
Dr S. Madokoro
Dr R. Matsubara
Dr K. Misaki
Dr I. Murata
Dr M. Oomori

Kyushu University, Fukuoka
Dr K. Hirata
*Dr H. Ninomiya
Dr T. Saito
Dr T. Tanaka

Fukushima Medical College, Fukushima
*Dr M. Kaneko
Dr K. Takahagi

Hirosaki University, Hirosaki
*Dr Y. Fukushima
Dr K. Hashimoto
Dr S. Kaneko
Dr K. Otani
Dr F. Saito
Dr H. Tasaki
Dr H. Yabe
Dr I. Yoshimura

Hiroshima University Hospital, Hiroshima
Dr Y. Ishida
*Dr M. Osada

Teikyo University, Ichihara Hospital, Ichihara
Dr M. Hasegawa
Dr R. Hayashi
Dr K. Hoshino
Dr M. Ikeda
Dr Y. Kim
Ms M. Matsumori
Dr T. Nemoto
*Dr T. Takahashi
Dr T. Takeuchi

Kanazawa University Hospital, Kanazawa
Dr H. Arai
Dr T. Asano
Dr T. Fukushima
Dr H. Hasegawa
Dr I. Jibiki
Dr H. Kido
Dr Y. Kiyota
Dr K. Kosaka
Dr Y. Koyama
Dr T. Maeda
Dr K. Miyazu
Dr K. Nakagawa
Dr H. Sakamoto
Dr T. Sumiyoshi
Dr K. Terai
Dr K. Urata

Dr K. Urasaki
Dr K. Ueno
*Dr N. Yamaguchi
Dr M. Yuasa

Tokyo Jikeikai University, Kashiwa Hospital, Kashiwa
Ms M. Kan
*Dr H. Kasahara
Dr S. Kishita
Dr H. Nishimura
Dr K. Nukariya
Dr M. Onda
Dr T. Shinozaki

University of Occupational and Environmental Health, Kitakyushu
Dr O. Ohmori
Dr T. Shiratsuchi
*Dr R. Yoshimura

Kurume University School of Medicine, Kurume
Dr Y. Ida
Dr T. Kotorii
Dr H. Mukasa
Dr J. Nakamura
*Dr Y. Nakazawa
Dr T. Sakamoto
Dr K. Takamuki
Dr S. Tsujimaru

Kyoto University, Kyoto
Dr S. Hamagaki
Dr Y. Inoue
Dr N. Marui
*Dr K. Nakayama
Dr A. Okae
Dr T. Yamashita

Miyazaki Medical College, Miyazaki
Dr O. Arakawa
Dr K. Hara
*Dr T. Ikeda

Kochi Medical School, Nangoku
Dr H. Hashizume
*Dr S. Inoue
Dr H. Sato

Hyogo College of Medicine, Nishinomiya
Dr K. Hori
Dr E. Hashiyama
Dr S. Hayashi
Dr S. Ikegami
Dr B. Iwamoto
Dr N. Kawasaki
Dr S. Komai
Dr H. Makihara
Dr M. Matsui
Dr K. Miki
Dr M. Miyamoto
*Dr K. Miyoshi
Dr Y. Morita
Dr Y. Nakai
Dr M. Sato
Dr Y. Shinoda
Dr S. Takauchi
Dr T. Takeda
Dr K. Tankiguchi
Dr S. Yamauchi
Dr A. Yoshikawa

Medical College of Oita, Oita
Dr J. Ando
*Dr I. Fujii
Dr N. Hasama
Dr J. Ihara
Dr H. Naganuma
Dr T. Yanagisawa

Okayama University Medical School, Okayama
Dr K. Akiyama
*Dr Y. Fujiwara

University of the Ryuku Hospital, Okinawa
Dr N. Kunimoto

Dr H. Nakamata
Dr H. Nakamoto
*Dr C. Ogura
Dr T. Uema
Dr K. Yamamoto

Shiga University of Medical Sciences, Ootsu
Ms R. Atsukawa
Dr K. Daimon
Dr K. Hanada
Mr H. Iida
Dr K. Ikemoto
Dr N. Kato
Dr T. Kato
Dr H. Kanai
Dr T. Noguchi
Dr K. Satoh
Dr T. Shioiri
Dr M. Shibasaki
Dr T. Someya
*Dr S. Takahashi

Kinki University, Osaka
*Dr M. Hanada
Dr T. Kusube
Dr A. Okada
Dr D. Takahashi
Dr H. Tazoe
Dr K. Yamaguchi
Dr T. Yokouchi

Osaka University Medical School, Osaka
Dr H. Sato
Dr A. Sekiyama
*Dr A. Yamamoto

Kitasato University, Sagamihara
Dr T. Arai
Dr J. Ishigooka
Dr T. Kasahara
Dr Y. Oguchi
*Dr Y. Ohtani

Hokkaido University, Sapporo
Dr K. Denda
Dr T. Kasahara
*Dr I. Yamashita

Keio University, Tokyo
*Dr M. Asai
Dr S. Kanba
Dr H. Kashima
Dr M. Mizuno
Dr A. Nishizono-Maher
Dr Y. Ono
Dr G. Yagi

Showa University, Tokyo
Dr F. Arakawa
Dr T. Hashimoto
Dr U. Inamoto
*Dr K. Kamijima
Dr M. Kawai
Dr N. Sakanishi
Dr I. Tadama

Tokyo Medical College Hospital, Tokyo
Dr S. Hikiba
Dr R. Ikeda
Dr M. Kato
Dr S. Koretsune
Dr T. Maruta
Dr S. Nagura
Dr N. Sakaue
*Dr M. Shimiz

Tokyo Medical and Dental University, Tokyo
Dr T. Kojima
Dr M. Matsuura
Dr Y. Okubo
*Dr M. Toru

Yamagata University Hospital, Yamagata
*Dr T. Nadaoka
Dr T. Tanaka

Field trial centres reporting to Oxford, England

Coordinating centre

Department of Psychiatry, Oxford University Hospital, Oxford
*Dr M. Gelder

Reporting centres

Czech Republic
Charles University, Hradec Kralove
*Dr M. Zaplatalek

Postgraduate Medical and Pharmaceutical Institute, Prague
Dr J. Beran
Dr K. Chromy
Dr K. Dusek
Dr D. Friedlova
Dr M. Hessler
Dr A. Janik
Dr N. Kubickova
Dr P. Pavlovsky
Dr P. Popov
*Dr P. Smolik

Prague Psychiatric Centre, Prague
Dr P. Baudis
Dr E. Bendova
Dr M. Benes
Dr I. Klar
*Dr D. Seifertova

England
Children's Hospital, Birmingham
*Dr R. Harrington
Dr P. Vostanis

Queen Elizabeth Psychiatric Hospital, Birmingham
Dr M. Baxter
Dr D. Clarke

*Dr J. Corbett
*Dr S. Cumella
Dr J. Langton
Dr V. Prasher
Dr A. Roy
Dr M. Roy
Dr K. Thinn

Ida Darwin Hospital, Cambridge
Dr S.J. Barnett
*Dr G. O'Brien

General Infirmary at Leeds, Leeds
*Dr I. Berg
Dr C. Lucas
Dr R. Sims
Dr A. Worrall

Department of Psychiatry, University of Leicester, Leicester
*Dr T.S. Brugha

Mossley Hill Hospital, Liverpool
Dr J. Copeland
Dr P. Saunders
*Dr K.C.M. Wilson

Guy's Hospital, London
*Dr T. Craig
Dr K. Sutherby

Institute of Psychiatry, London
*Dr A. Mann
Dr M. Phelan
Dr J. Rutherford

Maudsley Hospital, London
Dr G.O. Donoghue
Dr G.F.M. Russell
Dr J. Rutherford
Dr U. Schmidt
Dr J. Tiller
*Dr J. Treasure

MRC Social and Community Psychiatric Unit, Institute of Psychiatry, University of London, London
*Dr P. Bebbington

St Bartholomew's Hospital, London
*Dr P.D. White

St Charles Hospital, London
Dr P. Duke
Ms F. Henderson
Dr S. Merson
*Dr P. Tyrer

St Mary's Hospital, London
Dr D. Baldwin
Dr D. Montgomery
*Dr S.A. Montgomery

Worcester Royal Infirmary, Worcester
*Dr G. Milner
Dr R. Sheen
Dr J. Tarry
Dr G. Wainscott

Ireland

St Loman's Hospital, Dublin
Dr B. Murphy
*Dr A. O'Grady Walsh
Dr D. Walsh

Turkey

Hacettepe University, Ankara
Dr M. Gürsoy
*Dr A. Göğüş
Dr I. Kaplan
Dr R. Özbayrak
Dr G. Özgen
Dr M. Rezaki
Dr A. Sağduyu
Dr B. Uluğ
Dr A. Uluşahin

Field trial centres reporting to Aarhus, Denmark

Coordinating centre

Psychiatric University Hospital in Aarhus, Department B, Risskov
*Dr A. Bertelsen
Dr R. Licht
Dr S. Straarup

Reporting centres

Denmark

Psychiatric University Hospital in Aarhus, Department D, Risskov
*Dr N.C. Gulman

Hvidovre Hospital, Copenhagen
*Dr M. Kastrup
Dr K. Maarbjerg
Dr E. Simonsen

Frederiksberg Hospital, Frederiksberg, Copenhagen
Dr O. Jørgensen
*Dr J.K. Larsen
Dr K. Olafsson
Dr H. Raben
Dr H.R. Vinding

Randers Centralsygehus, Randers
Dr T. Mathiesen
*Dr J.A. Nielsen

Israel

"Talbieh" Mental Health Centre, Jerusalem
Dr R. Aronzon
Dr P. Brown
Dr N. Cividali
Dr R. Durst
Dr M. Fliman
*Dr Y. Ginath
Dr E. Perl
Dr M. Ritsner
Dr K.J. Rubin
Dr H. Schonfeld
Dr L. Zilberman

The Gehah Psychiatric Hospital, Petah-Tiqua, Tel-Aviv
Dr Z. Marom
*Dr H. Munitz
Dr G. Retzoni
Dr J. Sever

Poland

Department of Psychiatry I, Institute of Psychiatry and Neurology, Sobieskiego, Warsaw
Dr A. Chojnowska
Dr I. Stanikovska
*Dr J. Wciórka

Department of Psychiatry IV, Institute of Psychiatry and Neurology, Brodno General Hospital, Warsaw
Dr A. Bialyszewski
*Dr A. Piotrowski
Dr M. Zaluska

Romania

Psychiatric Department, Faculty of Medicine, University of Timisoara, Timisoara
Dr M. Dehelean
Dr P. Dehelean
Dr M. Ienciu
*Dr M. Lazarescu
Dr O. Nicoara
Dr F. Romosan

Field trial centres reporting to Rockville, MD, USA

Coordinating centre

Division of Clinical Research, National Institute of Mental Health, Rockville
*Dr G. Regier

Reporting centres

Canada

Alberta Hospital, Edmonton
Dr M. Cummins
*Dr P. Flor-Henry
Dr D. Spaner
Dr A. Van Zyl

London Psychiatric Hospital, London
Dr A. Hinsberger
Dr D. Mazmanian
*Dr E. Persad
Dr V. Sharma

University Hospital of Western Ontario, London
*Dr H. Merskey
Dr P. Monahar
Dr R. Manchanda

Douglas Hospital Research Center, Montreal
Dr S.K. Ahmed
*Dr H.E. Lehmann
Dr J. Martial
Dr A. Skorzewsky

Republic of Korea

Kyung-Pook National University Hospital, Daegu
Dr Kim Hyun-Joon
*Dr Lee Zuk-Nae

Asan Medical Center, Seoul
Dr Han Oh-Su
Dr Kim Chang Yoon
*Dr Lee Chul
Dr Park In Ho

Gyeongsang National University, Chinju
*Dr Hahn Kyu Hee
Dr Woo Sung Il

Hallym University Hospital, Seoul
Dr Ahn Dong Hyun
*Dr Ahn Seok Cheol

Kangdong Sacred Heart Hospital, Seoul
Dr Park Yu Moon
*Dr Suk Jae Ho
Dr Yeon Byeong Kil

Kangnam St Mary's Hospital, Seoul
Dr Chae Young Lae
Dr Choi Bo Moon
Dr Lee Chul
*Dr Paik In Ho

Seoul National Mental Hospital, Seoul
Dr Baek Ki-Cheong
*Dr Kwack Young Sook

Seoul National University Hospital (for adult patients), Seoul
Dr Jeong Do-Un
Dr Kim Do-Kwan
Dr Kim Yong-Sik
Dr Kwon Jun-Soo
*Dr Rhi Bou-Young
Dr Suh Tong Woo

Seoul National University Hospital (for paediatric patients), Seoul
Dr Cho Soo-Churl
Dr Choi Jin Sook
*Dr Hong Kang E.M.

Inje University Hospital, Seoul
*Dr Lee Jeong Ho
Dr Lee Ki-Cheol

Soonchunhyang University Hospital, Seoul
*Dr Han Sun Ho
Dr Jung Han Yong
Dr Kim Seung Hyun

Yonsei University, Seoul
Dr Jun Jie Hong
Dr Kim Young Shin
Dr Lee Bum Yong
Dr Lee Hee Sang
*Dr Lee Ho Young
Dr Lee Joo-Hun
Dr Lee Man-Hong
Dr Oh Byoung Hoon
Dr Shin Eui Jin

United States of America

McLean Hospital, Belmont
*Dr S. Frazier
Dr K. Phillips
Dr J. Samson

Baylor College of Medicine, Houston
Dr H. Clay
Dr F. Dereboy
*Dr N. Gokcebay
Dr M. Hirschkowitz
*Dr I. Karacan

Western Psychiatric Institute and Clinic, Pittsburgh
Dr S. Blaha
Dr J. Eichhorn
Dr M. Landy
*Dr R. Pary
Dr J.C. Rogers
Dr J.E. Salta

Washington University School of Medicine, St Louis
Dr T.S. Early
*Dr A. Janca

Field trial centres reporting to Shanghai, China

Coordinating centre

Shanghai Mental Health Centre, Shanghai
Dr Shi Shen-xun
Dr Xia Mei-lan
*Dr Xu Tao-yuan
Dr Zhang Yong-hua
Dr Zhu Zi-qing

Reporting centres

Hunan Medical University, Changsha
Dr Li Ling-jiang
*Dr Yang De-sen

West China Medical University, Chengdu
Dr Guo Lan-ting
Dr Li Tao
Dr Lin Pei-yi
*Dr Liu Xie-he
Dr Sun Xue-li
Dr Yang Yan-chun
Dr Ye Lu

Nanjing Institute of Child Mental Health, Nanjing
Dr Luo Shuo-jun
*Dr Tao Guo-tai
Dr Wang Ming-jie
Dr Zhang Ju-feng

Field trial centres reporting to Wellington, New Zealand

Coordinating centre

Wellington Hospital, Wellington
Dr J. Crawshaw
Dr P.M. Ellis
*Dr G.W. Mellsop
Dr N. Mendis
Dr G. Purdie
Dr C.S. Thomas

Reporting centre

University of Otago, Dunedin
Dr N. Raja
*Dr G.S. Ungvari

Index

Notes: For those entries marked # see List of categories for additional fourth, fifth or sixth character.

The letters NEC stand for "not elsewhere classified"; they are added after terms classified to residual categories, as a warning that specified forms of the conditions are classified differently.

Inclusion terms for all categories may be found in *Clinical descriptions and diagnostic guidelines.*

Page numbers are shown in italics.

Abuse (of) (*see also* Use, harmful)
– analgesics F55.2 *122*
– antacids F55.3 *122*
– antidepressants F55.0 *122*
– – tetracyclic F55.0 *122*
– – tricyclic F55.0 *122*
– aspirin F55.2 *122*
– diuretics F55.8 *122*
– hormones F55.5 *122*
– laxatives F55.1 *122*
– monamine oxidase inhibitors F55.0 *122*
– non-dependence-producing substances F55.– *121*
– – specified NEC F55.8 *122*
– paracetamol F55.2 *122*
– phenacetin F55.2 *122*
– specific folk remedies F55.6 *122*
– specific herbal remedies F55.6 *122*
– steroids F55.5 *122*
– vitamins F55.4 *122*

Adjustment disorder (*see* Disorder, adjustment)

Aerophagy, psychogenic F45.31 ***108***

Agoraphobia
– with panic disorder F40.01 *92*
– without panic disorder F40.00 *92*

Alcohol (*see also* Psychoactive substance-induced)
– intoxication
– – acute F10.0 # *49*
– – pathological F10.07 *50*
– withdrawal F10.3 *58*

Alzheimer's disease, dementia in F00.– # *31*
– atypical type F00.2 # *33*
– early onset F00.0 # *32*
– late onset F00.1 # *33*
– mixed type F00.2 # *33*

Amnesia, dissociative F44.0 *102*

Amnesic syndrome (*see* Syndrome, amnesic)

Anaesthesia and sensory loss, dissociative F44.6 *104*

Anankastic personality disorder F60.5 *127*

Anorexia nervosa F50.0 *112*
– atypical F50.1 *112*

Anxiety, episodic paroxysmal F41.0 *94*

Anxiety disorder (*see* Disorder, anxiety)

Anxious personality disorder F60.6 *128*

Aphasia, acquired, with epilepsy F80.3 *143*

Asperger's syndrome F84.5 *153*

Asthenia, neurocirculatory F45.30 *108*

Attachment disorder of childhood (*see* Disorder, attachment)

Attention deficit *157*

Autism
- atypical F84.1 *149*
- – in age of onset F84.10 *150*
- – in age of onset and symptomatology F84.12 *150*
- – in symptomatology F84.11 *150*
- childhood F84.0 *147*

Aversion, sexual F52.10 ***117***

Avoidant personality disorder F60.6 ***128***

Bipolar affective disorder (*see* Disorder, bipolar affective)

Borderline personality disorder F60.31 ***126***

Bulimia nervosa F50.2 ***113***
- atypical F50.3 *113*

Cannabinoid (*see also* Psychoactive substance-induced)
- intoxication, acute F12.0 # *51*
- withdrawal state F12.3 # *59*

Cataplexy G47.4 (*see* ICD-10, p. 409)

Caffeine (*see* Stimulants)

Cluttering F98.6 ***171***

Cocaine (*see also* Psychoactive substance-induced)
- intoxication, acute F14.0 # *53*
- withdrawal state F14.3 # *60*

Compulsive acts F42.1 ***98***

Conduct disorder (*see* Disorder, conduct)

Conversion disorder (*see* Disorder, dissociative)

Convulsions, dissociative F44.5 ***103***

Creutzfeldt–Jakob disease, dementia in F02.1 # ***35***

Cyclothymia F34.0 *87*

Da Costa's syndrome F45.30 *108*

Delirium (of) (in) F05.– *38*
– acute intoxication F1*x*.03 *49*
– not superimposed on dementia F05.0 *39*
– specified NEC F05.8 *39*
– superimposed on dementia F05.1 *39*
– withdrawal state F1x.4 *61*

Delusional disorder (*see* Disorder, delusional)

Dementia (in) (due to) F03 # *37*
– Alzheimer's disease F00.– # *31*
– – atypical type F00.2 # *33*
– – early onset F00.0 # *32*
– – late onset F00.1 # *33*
– – mixed type F00.2 # *33*
– Creutzfeldt–Jakob disease F02.1 # *35*
– disease specified NEC F02.8 # *37*
– human immunodeficieny virus [HIV] disease F02.4 # *37*
– Huntington's chorea (disease) F02.2 # *36*
– multi-infarct F01.1 # *34*
– Parkinson's disease F02.3 # *36*
– Pick's disease F02.0 # *35*
– psychoactive substances F1*x*.73 *63*
– vascular (of) F01.– # *33*
– – acute onset F01.0 # *34*
– – mixed cortical and subcortical F01.3 # *34*
– – specified NEC F01.8 # *35*
– – subcortical F01.2 # *34*

Dependence (*see* Syndrome, dependence)

Dependent personality disorder F60.7 *128*

Depersonalization–derealization syndrome F48.1 *110*

Depression, post-schizophrenic F20.4 # *67*

Depressive
– disorder (*see* Disorder, depressive)
– episode (*see* Episode, depressive)

Derealization syndrome F48.1 ***110***

Desire, sexual, lack or loss F52.0 ***117***

Developmental disorder (*see* Disorder, developmental)

Dhat syndrome F48.8 ***110, 178***

Diarrhoea, psychogenic F45.32 ***108***

Disease, dementia in
– Alzheimer's F00.– # *31*
– Creutzfeldt–Jakob F02.1 # *35*
– Huntington's F02.2 # *36*
– Parkinson's F02.3 # *36*
– Pick's F02.0 # *35*

Disorder (of)
– adjustment F43.2 *100*
– – anxiety and depressive reaction (mixed) F43.22 *101*
– – brief depressive reaction F43.20 *101*
– – prolonged depressive reaction F43.21 *101*
– – with mixed disturbance of emotions and conduct F43.25 *101*
– – with other specified predominant symptoms F43.28 *101*
– – with predominant disturbance of conduct F43.24 *101*
– – with predominant disturbance of other emotions F43.23 *101*
– affective (*see also* Disorder, mood)
– – residual, due to psychoactive substances F1*x*.72 *63*
– – seasonal *173*
– anxiety
– – and depressive, mixed F41.2 *97*
– – generalized F41.1 *95*
– – – of childhood F93.80 *164*
– – mixed F41.3 *97*
– – phobic F40.– *91*
– – – of childhood F93.1 *163*
– – – specified NEC F40.8 *94*

Disorder (of) (*continued*)
– anxiety (*continued*)
– – separation, of childhood F93.0 *162*
– – social, of childhood F93.2 *163*
– – specified NEC F41.– *94*
– arithmetical skills, specific F81.2 *146*
– articulation (speech), specific F80.0 *142*
– attachment, of childhood
– – disinhibited F94.2 *167*
– – reactive F94.1 *166*
– behavioural (*see* Disorder, mental and behavioural)
– bipolar II *173*
– bipolar (affective) F31.– *79*
– – current episode
– – – hypomanic F31.0 *79*
– – – manic
– – – – with psychotic symptoms F31.2 *79*
– – – – – mood-congruent F31.20 *80*
– – – – – mood-incongruent F31.21 *80*
– – – – without psychotic symptoms F31.1 *79*
– – – mild or moderate depression
– – – – with somatic syndrome F31.31 *80*
– – – – without somatic syndrome F31.30 *80*
– – – mixed F31.6 *81*
– – – severe depression
– – – – with psychotic symptoms F31.5 *80*
– – – – – mood-congruent F31.50 *81*
– – – – – mood-incongruent F31.51 *81*
– – – – without psychotic symptoms F31.4 *80*
– – in remission (currently) F31.7 *81*
– – organic F06.31 *42*
– – rapid cycling *173*
– – single manic episode F30.– *77*
– – specified NEC F31.8 *81*
– body dysmorphic F45.2 *106*
– childhood disintegrative, specified NEC F84.3 *151*
– cognitive, mild F06.7 *42*
– conduct F91.– *157*
– – confined to the family context F91.0 *160*
– – depressive F92.0 *161*
– – hyperkinetic F90.1 *157*
– – oppositional defiant F91.3 *161*

– – socialized F91.2 *160*
– – unsocialized F91.1 *160*
– – with depressive disorder (F30–F39) F92.0 *161*
– – with emotional disorder (F93.–) F92.8 *161*
– – with neurotic disorder (F40–F48) F92.8 *161*
– conversion F44.– *102*
– – mixed F44.7 *104*
– – specified NEC F44.8 *104*
– culture-specific *176*
– delusional F22.0 *70*
– – induced F24 *73*
– – persistent F22.– *70*
– – – specified NEC F22.8 *70*
– depressive
– – organic F06.32 *42*
– – recurrent F33.– *85*
– – – brief F38.10 *90*
– – – current episode
– – – – mild F33.0 *85*
– – – – – with somatic syndrome F33.01 *85*
– – – – – without somatic syndrome F33.00 *85*
– – – – moderate F33.1 *86*
– – – – – without somatic syndrome F33.10 *86*
– – – – – with somatic syndrome F33.11 *86*
– – – – severe
– – – – – with psychotic symptoms F33.3 *86*
– – – – – – mood-congruent F33.30 *86*
– – – – – – mood-incongruent F33.31 *86*
– – – – – without psychotic symptoms F33.2 *86*
– – – in remission F33.4 *86*
– – – specified NEC F33.8 *87*
– – single episode F32.– *81*
– developmental (specific) F80–F89
– – arithmetical skills F81.2 *146*
– – language F80.– *142*
– – – specified NEC F80.8 *144*
– – mixed, specific F83 *147*
– – motor function F82 *147*
– – pervasive F84.– *147*
– – psychological F89 *154*
– – scholastic skills F81.– *144*
– – – mixed F81.3 *146*

Disorder (of) (*continued*)
– developmental (specific) (*continued*)
– – specified NEC F88 *154*
– – speech F80.– *142*
– – – specified NEC F80.8 *144*
– dissociative F44.– *102*
– – mixed F44.7 *104*
– – motor F44.4 *103*
– – specified NEC F44.88 *104*
– – transient, in childhood and adolescence F44.82 *104*
– eating F50.– *112*
– – specified NEC F50.8 *113*
– emotional, of childhood F93.– *162*
– – specified NEC F93.8 *164*
– feeding, of infancy and childhood F98.2 *170*
– gender identity F64.– *133*
– – of childhood F64.2 *134*
– – specified NEC F64.8 *135*
– habit and impulse F63.– *132*
– – specified NEC F63.8 *133*
– hyperkinetic F90.– *155*
– – conduct F90.1 *157*
– language, developmental F80.– *142*
– – expressive F80.1 *142*
– – receptive F80.2 *143*
– manic, organic F06.30 *42*
– maturation, sexual F66.0 *138*
– mental and behavioural (due to) F99 *172*
– – alcohol-induced F10.– *63*
– – brain damage and dysfunction F06.– *39*
– – – specified NEC F06.8 *44*
– – caffeine-induced F15.– *48*
– – cannabinoid-induced F12.– *48*
– – cocaine-induced F14.– *48*
– – hallucinogen-induced F16.– *48*
– – hypnotic-induced F13.– *48*
– – in puerperium F53.– *120*
– – – mild F53.0 *121*
– – – specified NEC F53.8 *121*
– – – severe F53.1 *121*
– – multiple drug-induced F19 – *48*

– – opioid-induced F11.– *48*
– – organic F09 *47*
– – physical disease F06.– *39*
– – – specified NEC F06.8 *44*
– – psychoactive substance-induced F19.– *48*
– – sedative-induced F13.– *48*
– – specified NEC F1*x*.8 *63*
– – stimulant-induced F15.– *48*
– – symptomatic F09 *47*
– – tobacco-induced F17.– *48*
– – volatile solvent-induced F18.– *48*
– mild cognitive F06.7 *42*
– – associated with a physical disorder F06.71 *43*
– – not associated with a physical disorder F06.70 *43*
– mood [affective] F30–F39 *77*
– – organic F06.3 *42*
– – persistent F34.– *87*
– – – specified NEC F34.8 *89*
– – recurrent, specified NEC F38.1 *90*
– – single episode, specified NEC F38.0 *89*
– – specified NEC F38.– *89*
– motor function, specific F82 *147*
– neurotic, specified NEC F48.– *109*
– obsessive–compulsive F42.– *97*
– – specified NEC F42.8 *98*
– oppositional defiant F91.3 *161*
– organic F09 *47*
– – anxiety F06.4 *42*
– – asthenic F06.6 *42*
– – bipolar F06.31 *42*
– – catatonic F06.1 *40*
– – delusional [schizophrenia-like] F06.2 *41*
– – depressive F06.32 *42*
– – dissociative F06.5 *42*
– – emotionally labile [asthenic] F06.6 *42*
– – manic F06.30 *42*
– – mental F09 *47*
– – mixed affective F06.33 *42*
– – mood [affective] F06.3 *42*
– – personality F07.0 *44*
– – schizophrenia-like F06.2 *41*

Disorder (of) (*continued*)
– overactive, with mental retardation and stereotyped movements F84.4 *152*
– pain, persistent somatoform F45.4 *108*
– panic F41.0 *94*
– – moderate F41.00 *95*
– – severe F41.01 *95*
– – with agoraphobia F40.01 *92*
– personality F60.– *123*
– – anankastic F60.5 *127*
– – and behaviour (adult) F69 *139*
– – – organic, due to brain disease, damage and dysfunction F07.– *44*
– – – specified NEC F68.– *138*
– – anxious F60.6 *128*
– – avoidant F60.6 *128*
– – borderline F60.31 *126*
– – dependent F60.7 *128*
– – dissocial F60.2 *125*
– – emotionally unstable
– – – borderline type F60.31 *126*
– – – impulsive type F60.30 *126*
– – histrionic F60.4 *127*
– – mixed type F61.0 *129*
– – multiple F44.81 *104*
– – narcissistic *174*
– – negativistic *174*
– – obsessive–compulsive F60.5 *127*
– – organic F07.0 *44*
– – paranoid F60.0 *124*
– – passive–aggressive *174*
– – schizoid F60.1 *125*
– – schizotypal F21 *69*
– pervasive developmental F84.– *147*
– – specified NEC F84.8 *154*
– phobic anxiety F40.– *91*
– – of childhood F93.1 *163*
– – specified NEC F40.8 *94*
– phonological, developmental F80.0 *142*
– possession F44.3 *102*
– post-traumatic stress F43.1 *99*
– psychosexual development F66.– *138*
– – specified NEC F66.8 *138*

– psychotic
– – acute
– – – polymorphic
– – – – with symptoms of schizophrenia F23.1 # *72*
– – – – without symptoms of schizophrenia F23.0 # *72*
– – – predominantly delusional F23.3 # *73*
– – – schizophrenia-like F23.2 # *72*
– – acute and transient F23.– *71*
– – – specified NEC F23.8 *73*
– – alcohol-induced F10.5 # *62*
– – cannabinoid-induced F12.5 # *62*
– – cocaine-induced F14.5 # *62*
– – hallucinogen-induced F16.5 # *62*
– – hypnotic-induced F13.5 # *62*
– – late-onset, psychoactive substance-induced F1*x*.75 *63*
– – multiple drug-induced F19.5 # *62*
– – – specified F1*x*.5 *62*
– – opioid-induced F11.5 # *62*
– – polymorphic, acute (*see* Disorder, psychotic, acute)
– – psychoactive substance-induced F1*x*.5 # *62*
– – residual or late-onset F1*x*.7 # *63*
– – – alcohol-induced F10.7 # *63*
– – – caffeine-induced F15.7 # *63*
– – – cannabinoid-induced F12.7 # *63*
– – – cocaine-induced F14.7 # *63*
– – – hallucinogen-induced F16.7 # *63*
– – – hypnotic-induced F13.7 # *63*
– – – multiple drug-induced F19.7 # *63*
– – – opioid-induced F11.7 # *63*
– – – psychoactive substance-induced F1*x*.7 # *63*
– – – sedative-induced F13.7 # *63*
– – – stimulant-induced NEC F15.7 # *63*
– – – tobacco-induced F17.7 # *63*
– – – volatile solvent-induced F18.7 # *63*
– – sedative-induced F13.5 # *62*
– – stimulant-induced NEC F15.5 # *62*
– – tobacco-induced F17.5 # *62*
– – volatile solvent-induced F18.5 # *62*
– reading, specific F81.0 *144*
– recurrent [affective] mood (*see* Disorder, mood)
– relationship, sexual F66.2 *138*

Disorder (of) (*continued*)
– schizoaffective F25.– # *74*
– – depressive type F25.1 # *75*
– – manic type F25.0 # *75*
– – mixed type F25.2 # *75*
– – specified NEC F25.8 # *75*
– scholastic skills, developmental (specific) F81.– *144*
– – mixed F81.3 *146*
– – specified NEC F81.8 *146*
– seasonal affective *173*
– sexual
– – desire, lack or loss F52.0 *117*
– – maturation F66.0 *138*
– – preference F65.– *135*
– – – specified NEC F65.8 *137*
– – relationship F66.2 *138*
– sibling rivalry F93.3 *164*
– sleep
– – nonorganic F51.– *114*
– – – specified NEC F51.8 *116*
– social functioning, of childhood and adolescence F94.– *166*
– – specified NEC F94.8 *167*
– somatization F45.0 *105*
– somatoform F45.– *105*
– – pain, persistent F45.4 *108*
– – specified NEC F45.8 *108*
– – undifferentiated F45.1 *106*
– specific (developmental) (of)
– – arithmetical skills F81.3 *146*
– – language F80.– *142*
– – mixed F83 *147*
– – motor function F82 *147*
– – personality F60.– *123*
– – reading F81.0 *144*
– – scholastic skills F81.– *144*
– – – mixed F81.3 *146*
– – speech F80.– *142*
– – – articulation F80.0 *142*
– – – phonological F80.0 *142*
– – spelling F81.1 *145*
– speech articulation, specific F80.0 *142*
– spelling, specific F81.1 *145*

– stress, post-traumatic F43.1 *99*
– tic F95.– *167*
– – chronic
– – – motor F95.1 *168*
– – – vocal F95.1 *168*
– – combined vocal and multiple motor F95.2 *168*
– – specified NEC F95.8 *168*
– – transient F95.0 *167*
– trance and possession F44.3 *102*

Dissocial personality disorder F60.2 *125*

Dissociative disorder (*see* Disorder, dissociative)

Disturbance (predominant) of
– activity and attention F90.0 *157*
– conduct in adjustment disorder F43.24 *101*
– emotions and conduct, mixed, in adjustment disorder F43.25 *101*
– emotions, specified NEC, in adjustment disorder F43.23 *101*

Dual-role transvestism F64.1 *134*

Dysfunction
– orgasmic F52.3 *118*
– sexual, not caused by organic disorder or disease F52.– *116*
– – specified NEC F52.8 *120*
– somatoform autonomic (of) F45.3 *107*
– – genitourinary system F45.34 *108*
– – heart and cardiovascular system F45.30 *108*
– – lower gastrointestinal tract F45.32 *108*
– – respiratory system F45.33 *108*
– – specified organ NEC F45.38 *108*
– – upper gastrointestinal tract F45.31 *108*

Dysmorphophobia F45.2 *106*

Dyspareunia, nonorganic F52.6 *120*

Dysthymia F34.1 *88*

Dysuria, psychogenic F45.34 *108*

Ejaculation, premature F52.4 ***119***

Elaboration of physical symptoms for psychological reasons F68.0 ***138***

Elective mutism F94.0 ***166***

Emotionally unstable personality disorder (*see* Disorder, personality)

Encopresis, nonorganic F98.1 # ***169***

Enuresis, nonorganic F98.0 ***169***
– diurnal F98.01 *169*
– nocturnal F98.00 *169*
– nocturnal and diurnal F98.02 *169*

Episode
– depressive F32.– *81*
– – mild F32.0 *82*
– – – with somatic syndrome F32.01 *83*
– – – without somatic syndrome F32.00 *83*
– – moderate F32.1 *83*
– – – with somatic syndrome F32.11 *83*
– – – without somatic syndrome F32.10 *83*
– – severe
– – – with psychotic symptoms F32.3 *84*
– – – – mood-congruent F32.30 *84*
– – – – mood-incongruent F32.31 *84*
– – – without psychotic symptoms F32.2 *84*
– – specified NEC F32.8 *85*
– hypomanic F30.0 *77*
– manic F30.– *77*
– – specified NEC F30.8 *79*
– – with psychotic symptoms F30.2 *78*
– – – mood-congruent F30.20 *79*
– – – mood-incongruent F30.21 *79*
– – without psychotic symptoms F30.1 *77*
– mixed affective F38.00 *89*
– mood [affective], single, specified NEC F38.0 *89*

Exhibitionism F65.2 ***136***

Factitious disorder F68.1 ***139***

Factors, psychological and behavioural, associated with disorders or diseases classified elsewhere F54 *121*

Failure of genital response F52.2 *118*

Feeding disorder of infancy and childhood F98.2 *170*

Feigning or intentional production of symptoms or disabilities (physical) (psychological) F68.1 *139*

Fetishism F65.0 *135*

Fetishistic transvestism F65.1 *136*

Fire-setting, pathological F63.1 *133*

Flashback
– post-traumatic *99*
– psychoactive substance-induced F1*x*.70 *63*

Fugue, dissociative F44.1 *102*

Gambling, pathological F63.0 *132*

Ganser's syndrome F44.80 *104*

Gender identity disorder (*see* Disorder, gender identity)

Genital response, failure of F52.2 *118*

Gilles de la Tourette's syndrome F95.2 *168*

Hallucinogen intoxication, acute F16.0 # (*see also* Psychoactive substance-induced) *54*

Hallucinosis, organic F06.0 *40*

Harmful use (*see* Use, harmful)

Hebephrenia F20.1 # *66*

Hiccough, psychogenic F45.31 *108*

Histrionic personality disorder F60.4 ***127***

HIV disease, dementia in F02.4 # ***37***

Huntington's chorea or disease, dementia in F02.2 # ***36***

Hyperkinetic disorder (*see* Disorder, hyperkinetic)

Hypersomnia, nonorganic F51.1 ***114***

Hyperventilation, psychogenic F45.33 ***108***

Hypnotic (*see also* Psychoactive substance-induced)
– intoxication, acute F13.0 # *52*
– withdrawal state F13.3 # *60*

Hypochondriasis F45.2 ***106***

Hypomania F30.0 ***77***

Induced delusional disorder F24 ***73***

Insomnia, nonorganic F51.0 ***114***

Intoxication, acute (due to)
– alcohol F10.0 # *49*
– cannabinoids F12.0 # *51*
– cocaine F14.0 # *53*
– hallucinogens F16.0 # *54*
– hypnotics F13.0 # *52*
– multiple drugs F19.0 # *56*
– opioids F11.0 # *51*
– psychoactive substances F1*x*.0 # *48*
– sedatives F13.0 # *52*
– stimulants NEC F15.0 # *53*
– tobacco F17.0 # *55*
– volatile solvents F18.0 # *55*

Irritable bowel syndrome, psychogenic F45.32 ***108***

Kleptomania F63.2 ***133***

Koro F48.8 ***110, 179***

Lack (or loss) of sexual
– desire F52.0 *117*
– enjoyment F52.11 *117*

Landau–Kleffner syndrome F80.3 ***143***

Language disorder, developmental F80.– ***142***

Latah F48.8 ***110, 180***

Loss of sexual desire F52.0 ***117***

Malingering Z76.5 (*see* ICD-10, p. 1162)

Mania F30.9 (*see also* Episode, manic) ***79***
– with psychotic symptoms F30.2 *78*
– – mood-congruent F30.20 *79*
– – mood incongruent F30.21 *79*
– without psychotic symptoms F30.1 *77*

Mental retardation (*see* Retardation, mental)

Micturition, increased frequency, psychogenic F45.34 ***108***

Mutism
– elective F94.0 *166*
– selective F94.0 *166*

Narcissistic personality disorder ***174***

Narcolepsy G47.4 (*see* ICD-10, p. 409)

Negativistic personality disorder ***174***

Neurasthenia F48.0 ***109***

Neurosis
– cardiac F45.30 *108*
– gastric F45.31 *108*

Nicotine intoxication, acute F17.0 (*see also* Tobacco) *55*

Nightmare F51.5 *116*

Night terrors F51.4 *115*

Obsessional
- rituals F42.1 *98*
- ruminations F42.0 *98*
- thoughts F42.0 *98*
- thoughts and acts, mixed F42.2 *98*

Obsessive–compulsive disorder (*see* Disorder, obsessive–compulsive)
- specified NEC F42.8 *98*
- personality disorder F60.5 *127*

Opioid (*see also* Psychoactive substance-induced)
- intoxication, acute F11.0 # *51*
- withdrawal state F11.3 # *59*

Orgasmic dysfunction F52.3 *118*

Orientation, sexual, egodystonic F66.1 *138*

Overeating associated with psychological disturbances, specified NEC F50.4 *113*

Paedophilia F65.4 *137*

Pain disorder, somatoform, persistent F45.4 *108*

Panic disorder F41.0 *94*

Paranoid
- personality disorder F60.0 *124*
- schizophrenia F20.0 # *66*

Parkinson's disease, dementia in F02.3 # *36*

Passive–aggressive personality disorder *174*

Pathological
– fire-setting F63.1 *133*
– gambling F63.0 *132*
– stealing F63.2 *133*

Persistent somatoform pain disorder F45.4 ***108***

Personality
– change (not due to brain damage or disease) (enduring) (after) F62.– *129*
– – bereavement F62.8 *132*
– – catastrophic experience F62.0 *129*
– – psychiatric illness F62.1 *131*
– – specified NEC F62.8 *132*
– – troublesome F61.1 *129*
– disorder (*see* Disorder, personality)

Phobia
– social F40.1 *92*
– specific (isolated) F40.2 *93*

Phobic anxiety disorder F40.– ***91***
– of childhood F93.1 *163*
– specified NEC F40.8 *94*

Physical symptoms, elaboration of, for psychological reasons F68.0 ***138***

Pica of infancy and childhood F98.3 ***170***

Pick's disease, dementia in F02.0 # ***35***

Possession disorder F44.3 ***102***

Postconcussional syndrome F07.2 ***46***

Postencephalitic syndrome F07.1 ***45***

Post-schizophrenic depression F20.4 # ***67***

Post-traumatic stress disorder F43.1 ***99***

Psychoactive substance-induced
– acute intoxication F1*x*.0 # *48*

Psychoactive substance-induced (*continued*)
– amnesic syndrome F1*x*.6 *62*
– cognitive impairment, persisting, specified NEC F1*x*.74 *63*
– dementia F1*x*.73 *63*
– dependence syndrome F1*x*.2 # *57*
– flashbacks F1*x*.70 *63*
– harmful use F1*x*.1 *56*
– intoxication, acute F1*x*.0 # *48*
– late-onset psychotic disorder F1*x*.75 *63*
– mental and behavioural disorder F1*x*.9 *63*
– – specified NEC F1*x*.8 *63*
– personality disorder F1*x*.71 *63*
– psychotic disorder F1*x*.5 # *62*
– residual disorder F1*x*.7 # *63*
– – affective F1*x*.72 *63*
– – behaviour F1*x*.71 *63*
– – personality F1*x*.71 *63*
– withdrawal state F1*x*.3 # *58*
– – with delirium F1*x*.4 # *61*

Psychosis, nonorganic F29 *76*

Puerperium, mental and behavioural disorders associated with (*see* Disorder, mental and behavioural)

Pyromania F63.1 *133*

Reaction
– acute stress F43.0 *98*
– – mild F43.00 *99*
– – moderate F43.01 *99*
– – severe F43.02 *99*
– depressive
– – and anxiety, mixed F43.22 *101*
– – brief F43.20 *101*
– – prolonged F43.21 *101*
– severe stress F43.– *98*
– – specified NEC F43.8 *101*

Reading disorder, specific F81.0 *144*

Retardation, mental
- mild F70 # *140*
- moderate F71 # *140*
- profound F73 # *140*
- severe F72 # *140*

Rett's syndrome F84.2 ***151***

Sadomasochism F65.5 ***137***

Schizoaffective disorder (*see* Disorder, schizoaffective)

Schizoid personality disorder F60.1 ***125***

Schizotypal disorder F21 ***69***

Schizophrenia F20.– # ***64***
- catatonic F20.2 # *67*
- hebephrenic F20.1 # *66*
- paranoid F20.0 # *66*
- residual F20.5 # *68*
- simple F20.6 # *68*
- specified NEC F20.8 # *69*
- undifferentiated F20.3 # *67*

Schizophrenia-like
- acute psychotic disorder (*see* Disorder, psychotic)
- disorder, organic F06.2 *41*

Seasonal affective disorder ***173***

Sedative (*see also* Psychoactive substance-induced)
- intoxication, acute F13.0 # *52*
- withdrawal state F13.3 # *60*

Selective mutism F94.0 ***166***

Separation anxiety disorder of childhood F93.0 ***162***

Sexual
- aversion F52.10 *117*
- desire, lack or loss F52.0 *117*

Sexual (*continued*)
– drive, excessive F52.7 *120*
– dysfunction, not caused by organic disorder or disease F52.– *116*
– enjoyment, lack of F52.11 *117*
– maturation disorder F66.0 *138*
– orientation, egodystonic F66.1 *138*
– preference disorder F65.– *135*
– – multiple F65.6 *137*
– – specified NEC F65.8 *137*
– relationship disorder F66.2 *138*

Sibling rivalry disorder F93.3 ***164***

Sleep
– disorder, non-psychogenic F51.9 *116*
– – specified NEC F51.8 *116*
– terrors F51.4 *115*

Sleep–wake schedule disorder, nonorganic F51.2 ***115***

Sleepwalking F51.3 ***115***

Social
– anxiety disorder of childhood F93.2 *163*
– phobia F40.1 *92*

Somatization disorder F45.0 ***105***

Somatoform
– autonomic dysfunction (*see* Dysfunction, somatoform autonomic)
– disorder (*see* Disorder, somatoform)

Somnambulism F51.3 ***115***

Specific disorder (of) (*see* Disorder, specific)

Spelling disorder, specific F81.1 ***145***

Speech articulation disorder, specific F80.0 ***142***

Stammering F98.5 ***171***

State, withdrawal
– alcohol F10.3 *58*
– – with delirium F10.4 # *61*
– caffeine F15. 3# *61*
– cannabinoids F12.3 # *59*
– cocaine F14.3 # *60*
– – with delirium F14.4 # *61*
– hallucinogens F16.3 # *61*
– – with delirium F16.4 # *61*
– hypnotics F13.3 # *60*
– – with delirium F13.4 # *61*
– multiple drugs F19.3 # *61*
– – with delirium F19.4 # *61*
– opioids F11.3 # *59*
– – with delirium F11.4 # *61*
– psychoactive substances F1*x*.3 # *58*
– – with delirium F1*x*.4 *61*
– sedatives F13.3 # *60*
– – with delirium F13.4 # *61*
– stimulants NEC F15.3 # *61*
– – – with delirium F15.4 # *61*
– tobacco F17.3 # *61*
– volatile solvents F18.3 # *61*
– – with delirium F18.4 # *61*

Stealing, pathological F63.2 ***133***

Stereotyped movement disorder F98.4 ***170***
– mixed F98.42 *171*
– non-self-injurious F98.40 *171*
– self-injurious F98.41 *171*

Stimulants (*see also* Psychoactive substance-induced)
– intoxication, acute F15.0 *53*
– withdrawal state F15.3 *61*

Stress
– reaction F43.– *98*
– – acute F43.0 *98*
– – – mild F43.00 *99*
– – – moderate F43.01 *99*
– – – severe F43.02 *99*

Stress *(continued)*
– reaction (*continued*)
– – specified NEC F43.8 *101*
– disorder, post-traumatic F43.1 *99*

Stupor, dissociative F44.2 ***102***

Stuttering F98.5 ***171***

Subnormality (*see* Retardation, mental)

Symptoms
– physical
– – elaboration of F68.0 *138*
– – feigning of F68.1 *139*
– – intentional production of F68.1 *139*
– psychological
– – feigning of F68.1 *139*
– – intentional production of F68.1 *139*

Syndrome
– alcohol withdrawal F10.3 # *58*
– amnesic
– – cannabinoid-induced F12.6 *62*
– – hallucinogen-induced F16.6 *62*
– – hypnotic-induced F14.6 *61*
– – multiple drug-induced F19.6 *61*
– – opioid-induced F11.6 *61*
– – organic (nonalcoholic) F04 *37*
– – psychoactive substance-induced NEC F19.6 *61*
– – sedative-induced F13.6 *61*
– – stimulant-induced NEC F15.6 *61*
– – volatile solvent-induced F18.6 *61*
– Asperger's F84.5 *153*
– Da Costa's F45.30 *108*
– dependence
– – alcohol F10.2 # *57*
– – caffeine F15.2 # *57*
– – cannabinoids F12.2 # *57*
– – cocaine F14.2 # *57*
– – hallucinogens F16.2 # *57*
– – hypnotics F13.2 *57*

– – multiple drugs F19.2 # *57*
– – opioids F11.2 # *57*
– – psychoactive substances NEC F19.2 # *57*
– – sedatives F13.2 # *57*
– – stimulants NEC F15.2 # *57*
– – tobacco F17.2 # *57*
– – volatile solvents F18.2 # *57*
– depersonalization–derealization F48.1 *110*
– dhat F48.8 *110*
– gas F45.32 *108*
– Ganser's F44.80 *104*
– irritable bowel, psychogenic F45.32 *108*
– Landau–Kleffner F80.3 *143*
– postconcussional F07.2 *46*
– postencephalitic F07.1 *45*
– Rett's F84.2 *151*
– somatic *82*
– Tourette's F95.2 *168*
– withdrawal (*see* State, withdrawal)

Tic (*see* Disorder, tic)

Tobacco (*see also* Psychoactive substance-induced)
– intoxication, acute F17.0 # *55*
– withdrawal state F17.3 # *61*

Tourette's syndrome F95.2 ***168***

Trance (and possession) disorder F44.3 ***102***

Transsexualism F64.0 ***133***

Transvestism
– dual-role F64.1 *134*
– fetishistic F65.1 *136*

Trichotillomania F63.3 ***133***

Use, harmful (nondependent)
– alcohol F10.1 *56*
– caffeine F15.1 *56*
– cannabinoids F12.1 *56*

Use, harmful (nondependent) (*continued*)
– cocaine F14.1 *56*
– hallucinogens F16.1 *56*
– hypnotics F13.1 *56*
– multiple drugs F19.1 *56*
– opioids F11.1 *56*
– psychoactive substances F1*x*.1 *56*
– sedatives F13.1 *56*
– stimulants NEC F15.1 *56*
– tobacco F17.1 *56*
– volatile solvents F18.1 *56*

Vaginismus, nonorganic F52.5 ***119***

Vascular dementia (*see* Dementia, vascular)

Vomiting associated with psychological disturbances, specified NEC F50.5 ***113***

Voyeurism F65.3 ***136***

Withdrawal state (*see* State, withdrawal)